CHRONIC LYMPHOCYTIC LEUKEMIA

DIET COOKBOOK

FOR BEGINNERS

Nourishing Recipes and Expert Guidance for Optimal Health and Immune Support

Kingsley Klopp

To show our appreciation for your purchase, we're delighted to offer you these special bonuses as a heartfelt thank you.

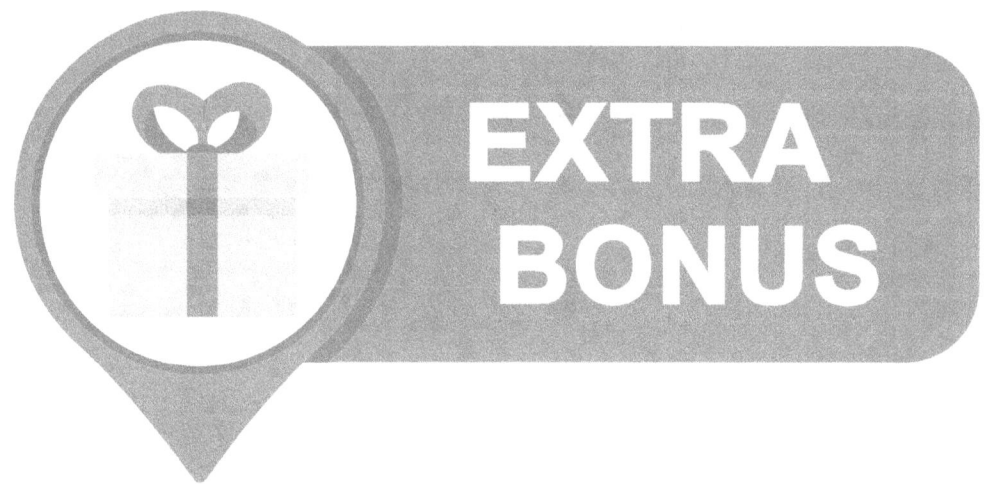

1. A Food Tracker Journal
2. Downloadable E-BOOK featuring full-color images of finished recipes

Table of Contents

Fish & Seafood Recipes.

Poultry Recipes

Soup and Stew Recipes

Important Note

As you set out on this culinary journey, we hope to provide you with not just recipes but a source of comfort, nourishment, and hope. Each dish is thoughtfully designed to support your health and well-being, with the goal of making your daily life a little easier and a lot more delicious. However, it's essential to remember that each person's experience with lymphocytic leukemia is unique, just as our dietary needs can vary significantly from one individual to another. While the recipes in this book offer a foundation for healthy eating, we encourage you to adjust the ingredients and portions to better suit your personal preferences and nutritional requirements.

Your body is your best guide, and it's important to listen to it. If you find yourself uncertain or need personalized advice on how to tailor these recipes to fit your health needs, please consult with your healthcare provider. They can offer guidance that ensures your diet complements your treatment plan and overall health strategy.

Additionally, please note that the nutritional information provided with each recipe is approximate. Variations in specific ingredients, brands, and portion sizes can affect the nutritional content. These figures are meant to serve as a general guide to help you make informed choices, but they are not exact calculations.

Furthermore, If our cookbook has brought joy to your kitchen and table, we'd be thrilled to hear about your experiences in an Amazon review. On the flip side, if you stumble upon any hiccups while exploring our recipes, don't hesitate to get in touch at **kloppkingsley@gmail.com.** We're here to support your cooking journey every step of the way.

Kingsley Klopp

Introduction

Imagine waking up each day, not to the vibrancy of sunrise but to the weight of chronic lymphocytic leukemia (CLL) on your shoulders. The diagnosis itself can be overwhelming, not to mention the journey that follows—the doctor visits, the treatments, and the unending search for ways to improve your quality of life. It's a path that demands resilience and hope, but also the right tools to help you along the way. That's where the **Chronic Lymphocytic Leukemia Diet Cookbook for Beginners** comes into play.

Welcome to a transformative culinary adventure designed specifically for those living with CLL. This isn't just another cookbook; it's a lifeline, a companion that brings together the science of nutrition and the art of cooking to support your health journey. Let's face it: living with CLL means making daily choices that affect your well-being, and food plays a monumental role in that equation. So, why focus on diet? Research has shown that what we eat can have a significant impact on our immune system, energy levels, and overall health. For those with CLL, a well-balanced diet is not just beneficial—it's essential. The right foods can help manage symptoms, boost your immune system, and provide the strength needed to combat the challenges of CLL. This cookbook is your guide to navigating these nutritional waters with confidence and ease. Each recipe within these pages is crafted to be simple, delicious, and most importantly, tailored to support the unique dietary needs of someone living with CLL. From nutrient-packed breakfasts to hearty dinners and refreshing snacks, you'll find a variety of dishes that cater to both your taste buds and your health.

But let's be real—this book is not about deprivation or bland, uninspiring meals. It's about discovering the joy of eating well, even when living with CLL. Imagine savoring a warm bowl of antioxidant-rich berry oatmeal to kickstart your day, or delighting in a colorful, immune-boosting salad for lunch. Picture ending your evening with a comforting, nutrient-dense soup that not only satisfies your hunger but also nourishes your body at a cellular level. In addition to providing mouth-watering recipes, this book is packed with practical advice on shopping for CLL-friendly ingredients, tips on meal planning, and strategies for maintaining a balanced diet even on your busiest days. You'll also find valuable information about specific foods to include in your diet, as well as those to avoid, all backed by the latest nutritional science.

Furthermore, this cookbook acknowledges the emotional journey that comes with living with CLL. Throughout the book, you'll find stories from others who have walked this path before you. Their experiences, challenges, and triumphs are shared to inspire and remind you that you are not alone. These narratives are woven into the fabric of this book to provide not just nutritional guidance, but also emotional support. It's important to note that while this cookbook offers a wealth of information and guidance, it is not a substitute for professional medical advice. Always consult with your healthcare provider before making any significant changes to your diet, especially when managing a condition like CLL. Each recipe includes approximate nutritional information, but remember, these values can vary based on specific ingredients and portion sizes.

So, here we are at the beginning of a journey that promises to be as rewarding as it is delicious. The "Chronic Lymphocytic Leukemia Diet Cookbook for Beginners" is more than a collection of recipes—it's a beacon of hope, a testament to the power of food as medicine, and a celebration of the resilience of the human spirit. Let's open the pages, tie on our aprons, and start cooking our way to better health and brighter days. Here's to nourishing your body, lifting your spirits, and finding joy in every bite.

Chapter 1: Understanding Chronic Lymphocytic Leukemia

What is Chronic Lymphocytic Leukemia?

Definition and Nature

Chronic Lymphocytic Leukemia is a type of cancer that originates in the bone marrow and affects the blood. Specifically, it targets a group of white blood cells called lymphocytes, which are crucial to the immune system. Unlike acute leukemia, CLL progresses slowly, often over many years, and primarily affects adults, with the majority of cases diagnosed in individuals over the age of 60. In CLL, the bone marrow produces too many lymphocytes that are not fully developed. These abnormal cells, called leukemia cells, accumulate over time and crowd out healthy blood cells, impairing the body's ability to fight infection and perform essential functions.

Historical Context

The history of CLL is intertwined with the broader story of leukemia and cancer research. The term "leukemia" was first coined in 1845 by Rudolf Virchow, a pioneering German pathologist, who observed an excessive number of white blood cells in the blood of affected patients. However, it wasn't until the early 20th century that CLL was distinguished as a specific type of leukemia. The mid-20th century marked significant advances in the understanding of leukemia. Researchers began to identify the genetic and molecular underpinnings of various types of leukemia, including CLL. This period saw the advent of cytogenetics, which allowed scientists to observe chromosomal abnormalities associated with leukemia. In CLL, the discovery of the 13q deletion, trisomy 12, and other genetic markers provided crucial insights into the disease's pathogenesis.

Development Over Time

The evolution of CLL research and treatment has been a story of hope and relentless pursuit of knowledge. Early treatments for CLL were limited and often ineffective, focusing primarily on symptom management rather than targeting the disease itself. The introduction of chemotherapy in the 1950s and 1960s provided some relief, but it was a blunt instrument, often accompanied by severe side effects. The 1990s and early 2000s marked a revolutionary period in CLL treatment. The development of targeted therapies, such as monoclonal antibodies (e.g., rituximab), offered more precise attacks on leukemia cells while sparing healthy cells. This era also saw the advent of immunotherapies and the exploration of stem cell transplants as potential cures. In recent years, the advent of next-generation sequencing and precision medicine has further transformed the landscape of CLL treatment. Scientists can now identify specific genetic mutations driving the disease in individual patients, allowing for personalized treatment plans. The approval of small molecule inhibitors, such as ibrutinib and venetoclax, has provided new hope for patients, significantly improving survival rates and quality of life.

Symptoms and Diagnosis

Symptoms of CLL

CLL symptoms can vary widely among individuals. Some people may not experience any symptoms for years, while others may notice changes in their health that prompt them to seek medical attention. The slow progression of CLL often means that symptoms develop gradually and can be subtle at first.

1. **Fatigue**
   - Description: One of the most common symptoms of CLL is persistent fatigue that doesn't improve with rest. This overwhelming tiredness can impact daily activities and overall quality of life.
   - Emotional Impact: Fatigue can be frustrating and debilitating, often leaving patients feeling powerless and disconnected from their usual routines.
2. **Frequent Infections**
   - Description: CLL weakens the immune system, making individuals more susceptible to infections. Common infections include respiratory infections, urinary tract infections, and skin infections.
   - Emotional Impact: Recurrent infections can be worrisome and exhausting, adding an extra layer of stress and anxiety for patients and their families.
3. **Swollen Lymph Nodes**
   - Description: Enlarged lymph nodes, often painless, can be felt in the neck, underarms, abdomen, or groin. This swelling occurs as leukemia cells accumulate in the lymphatic system.
   - Emotional Impact: Discovering swollen lymph nodes can be alarming and may lead to immediate concerns about the seriousness of the condition.
4. **Enlarged Spleen or Liver**
   - Description: The spleen and liver may enlarge due to the accumulation of leukemia cells, causing discomfort or a feeling of fullness in the upper left abdomen (spleen) or right side (liver).
   - Emotional Impact: Physical discomfort and visible changes can increase anxiety and affect daily comfort.
5. **Unintended Weight Loss**
   - Description: Significant weight loss without any change in diet or exercise habits can be a symptom of CLL.
   - Emotional Impact: Unexplained weight loss can be distressing and may lead to additional health concerns and self-image issues.

6. Night Sweats

- Description: Excessive sweating during the night, often drenching the bedclothes and sheets, is a common symptom of CLL.
- Emotional Impact: Night sweats can disrupt sleep patterns, leading to increased fatigue and emotional strain.

7. Fever

- Description: Unexplained fevers that come and go can be indicative of an underlying infection or the disease itself.
- Emotional Impact: Persistent fevers can cause worry and may necessitate frequent medical consultations.

8. Bruising and Bleeding

- Description: CLL can affect the blood's ability to clot, leading to easy bruising and prolonged bleeding from minor cuts.
- Emotional Impact: Bruising and bleeding can be visually alarming and may cause concerns about overall health and safety.

Diagnosis of CLL

Diagnosing CLL involves a series of tests and evaluations designed to confirm the presence of the disease and assess its extent. Early diagnosis is crucial for effective management and treatment.

1. **Medical History and Physical Examination**
   - Process: The diagnostic journey often begins with a detailed medical history and a physical examination. The doctor will ask about symptoms, duration, and any family history of blood disorders or cancers. During the physical examination, the doctor will check for swollen lymph nodes, an enlarged spleen, or liver.
   - Emotional Impact: Sharing symptoms and undergoing a physical exam can be a vulnerable experience, filled with anxiety about potential findings.

2. **Blood Tests**
   - Complete Blood Count (CBC): A CBC measures the levels of different blood cells. In CLL, there is usually an elevated number of lymphocytes.
   - Flow Cytometry: This test identifies specific markers on the surface of cells, helping to differentiate CLL from other types of leukemia.
   - Immunophenotyping: This technique helps to identify the specific subtype of leukemia cells.
   - Emotional Impact: Blood tests, while routine, can be stressful as patients await potentially life-altering results.

3. Bone Marrow Aspiration and Biopsy

- Process: If blood tests suggest CLL, a bone marrow aspiration and biopsy may be performed to confirm the diagnosis. This involves extracting a small amount of bone marrow, usually from the hip bone, to examine for leukemia cells.
- Emotional Impact: This procedure can be uncomfortable and anxiety-inducing, as it involves both physical discomfort and emotional stress over the results.

4. Imaging Tests

- CT Scans and Ultrasounds: Imaging tests can help determine if CLL has spread to other organs, such as the spleen, liver, or lymph nodes.
- Emotional Impact: The process of undergoing imaging tests can be daunting, and the anticipation of results can add to the emotional burden.

5. Genetic and Molecular Tests

- FISH (Fluorescence In Situ Hybridization): This test looks for specific genetic abnormalities in the leukemia cells that can influence prognosis and treatment options.
- PCR (Polymerase Chain Reaction): PCR can detect minimal residual disease by identifying tiny amounts of leukemia cells that might remain after treatment.
- Emotional Impact: Genetic testing can bring a mix of hope and fear, as results may impact treatment decisions and prognosis.

Treatment Options for Chronic Lymphocytic Leukemia (CLL)

Watchful Waiting (Active Surveillance)
- Description: For patients with early-stage CLL that is asymptomatic or slow-growing, doctors may recommend a strategy known as watchful waiting or active surveillance. This involves regular monitoring of the patient's condition without immediate treatment.
- Mechanism: Regular check-ups and blood tests are conducted to track the progression of the disease. Treatment begins only when symptoms appear or there are signs of disease progression.
- Emotional Impact: The concept of waiting can be emotionally challenging. Patients might experience anxiety and uncertainty, constantly wondering if or when the disease will progress. However, it can also be a relief to avoid the side effects of treatment for as long as possible.

Chemotherapy
- Description: Chemotherapy uses drugs to kill rapidly dividing cells, including cancer cells. It has been a cornerstone of CLL treatment for many years.
- Mechanism: Common chemotherapy drugs for CLL include fludarabine, cyclophosphamide, and chlorambucil. These drugs can be used alone or in combination with other therapies.
- Emotional Impact: Chemotherapy can be physically and emotionally taxing. Side effects such as nausea, hair loss, and fatigue can affect a patient's quality of life. The emotional strain of dealing with these side effects, along with the fear of treatment efficacy, can be significant.

Targeted Therapy
- Description: Targeted therapies are drugs designed to target specific molecules involved in the growth and survival of cancer cells.
- Mechanism:
  - Bruton's Tyrosine Kinase (BTK) Inhibitors: Drugs like ibrutinib and acalabrutinib block BTK, a protein that helps CLL cells survive and proliferate.
  - BCL-2 Inhibitors: Venetoclax targets the BCL-2 protein, which helps CLL cells avoid apoptosis (programmed cell death).
  - PI3K Inhibitors: Drugs like idelalisib inhibit PI3K, a protein involved in cell growth and survival.
- **Emotional Impact:** Targeted therapies often have fewer side effects than traditional chemotherapy, which can be a significant emotional relief. However, the high cost and the need for ongoing treatment can be sources of stress.

Immunotherapy

- Description: Immunotherapy harnesses the body's immune system to fight cancer. Monoclonal antibodies are a common form of immunotherapy used in CLL.
- Mechanism:
  - Monoclonal Antibodies: Rituximab, obinutuzumab, and ofatumumab target CD20, a protein on the surface of CLL cells, marking them for destruction by the immune system.
  - Checkpoint Inhibitors: These drugs help the immune system recognize and attack cancer cells by blocking proteins that prevent immune cells from attacking cancer.
- Emotional Impact: The prospect of using the body's own immune system to fight cancer can be empowering and hopeful for patients. However, side effects such as infusion reactions and increased risk of infections need to be managed, which can be challenging.

Stem Cell Transplantation

- Description: Stem cell transplantation (SCT), also known as bone marrow transplantation, involves replacing diseased bone marrow with healthy stem cells.
- Mechanism:
  - Autologous SCT: Uses the patient's own stem cells.
  - Allogeneic SCT: Uses stem cells from a donor, which can generate a new immune response against CLL cells.
- Emotional Impact: SCT can offer the possibility of long-term remission or cure but comes with significant risks and a long recovery period. The decision to undergo SCT can be fraught with fear and hope, as it involves intensive treatment and a lengthy hospital stay.

Clinical Trials

- Description: Participation in clinical trials can provide access to new and experimental treatments that are not yet widely available.
- Mechanism: Clinical trials test the safety and effectiveness of new drugs or treatment combinations. They follow strict protocols and are conducted in phases to ensure patient safety.
- Emotional Impact: Clinical trials can offer hope and a sense of contribution to future cancer research. However, the uncertainty of outcomes and the potential for unexpected side effects can be stressful.

Supportive Care and Palliative Treatment

- Description: Supportive care aims to improve quality of life by managing symptoms and side effects. Palliative care focuses on relief from the symptoms and stress of the disease.
- Mechanism: This can include medications for pain relief, treatments for infections, and therapies to manage fatigue and emotional support.
- Emotional Impact: Supportive and palliative care can significantly improve the emotional well-being of patients by addressing the physical and psychological challenges of living with CLL. It emphasizes the patient's comfort and quality of life, offering solace and support during difficult times.

Combination Therapies

- Description: Many patients receive a combination of treatments to maximize effectiveness.
- Mechanism: Combining chemotherapy with targeted therapy, or adding immunotherapy to a treatment regimen, can enhance the overall response to treatment.
- Emotional Impact: While combination therapies can be more effective, they can also increase the complexity and side effects of treatment. Patients may feel overwhelmed by the number of medications and the intensity of the treatment schedule.

Personalized Medicine

- Description: Advances in genetic testing and molecular biology have paved the way for personalized medicine, where treatment is tailored to the individual's genetic makeup and the specific characteristics of their disease.
- Mechanism: Genetic tests can identify specific mutations and markers that guide the selection of targeted therapies and predict response to treatment.
- Emotional Impact: Personalized medicine offers a beacon of hope, promising more effective and tailored treatments. However, the process of undergoing genetic testing and waiting for results can be anxiety-inducing.

Chapter 2: Nutritional Guidelines for CLL

Essential Nutrients for CLL Patients

Proteins
- Description: Proteins are the building blocks of the body, essential for the repair and growth of tissues. They play a crucial role in maintaining muscle mass, supporting the immune system, and aiding in recovery from illness or treatment.
- Sources: Lean meats (chicken, turkey), fish, eggs, dairy products, legumes (beans, lentils), nuts, and seeds.
- Benefits: Adequate protein intake can help prevent muscle wasting, support immune function, and enhance the body's ability to heal and recover from treatments.

Carbohydrates
- Description: Carbohydrates are the body's primary source of energy. They are essential for maintaining energy levels, especially during treatment, when the body's energy demands can increase.
- Sources: Whole grains (brown rice, quinoa, oats), fruits, vegetables, and legumes.
- Benefits: Complex carbohydrates provide sustained energy, help maintain blood sugar levels, and supply essential vitamins and minerals. They also support digestive health due to their fiber content.

Fats
- Description: Fats are vital for the absorption of fat-soluble vitamins (A, D, E, K) and provide a concentrated source of energy. Healthy fats also support brain function and reduce inflammation.
- Sources: Avocados, nuts, seeds, olive oil, fatty fish (salmon, mackerel), and flaxseeds.
- Benefits: Incorporating healthy fats into the diet can improve nutrient absorption, support brain health, and provide anti-inflammatory benefits, which are crucial for overall well-being.

Vitamins
1. Vitamin A
   - Role: Supports the immune system, vision, and skin health.
   - Sources: Carrots, sweet potatoes, spinach, kale, and fortified dairy products.
   - Benefits: Enhances immune function and helps maintain healthy skin and mucous membranes, which can be crucial for preventing infections.
2. Vitamin C
   - Role: An antioxidant that helps protect cells from damage and supports the immune system.
   - Sources: Citrus fruits (oranges, lemons), strawberries, bell peppers, broccoli, and kiwi.
   - Benefits: Boosts immune function, aids in the absorption of iron from plant-based foods, and helps in the repair of tissues.

3. Vitamin D
- Role: Essential for bone health and immune function.
- Sources: Sunlight exposure, fatty fish, fortified dairy products, and egg yolks.
- Benefits: Supports bone health, reduces the risk of infections, and may play a role in cancer prevention.

4. Vitamin E
- Role: An antioxidant that protects cells from damage and supports immune function.
- Sources: Nuts, seeds, spinach, and vegetable oils.
- Benefits: Protects cells from oxidative stress, supports immune health, and improves skin health.

5. Vitamin K
- Role: Essential for blood clotting and bone health.
- Sources: Leafy green vegetables (kale, spinach), broccoli, and Brussels sprouts.
- Benefits: Supports proper blood clotting and contributes to bone health, reducing the risk of fractures.

Minerals

1. Iron
  - Role: Crucial for the production of hemoglobin, which carries oxygen in the blood.
  - Sources: Red meat, poultry, fish, lentils, beans, and fortified cereals.
  - Benefits: Prevents anemia, reduces fatigue, and supports overall energy levels.

2. Calcium
  - Role: Essential for bone health and muscle function.
  - Sources: Dairy products, leafy green vegetables, fortified plant-based milks, and tofu.
  - Benefits: Maintains strong bones and teeth, supports muscle function, and reduces the risk of osteoporosis.

3. Magnesium
  - Role: Involved in over 300 biochemical reactions in the body, including energy production and muscle function.
  - Sources: Nuts, seeds, whole grains, legumes, and leafy green vegetables.
  - Benefits: Supports muscle and nerve function, maintains a healthy immune system, and regulates blood pressure.

4. Zinc
  - Role: Vital for immune function, wound healing, and DNA synthesis.
  - Sources: Meat, shellfish, legumes, seeds, nuts, and dairy products.
  - Benefits: Enhances immune response, promotes wound healing, and supports cell growth and repair.

Antioxidants

- Description: Antioxidants protect cells from damage caused by free radicals, which can contribute to cancer progression and other diseases.
- Sources: Fruits (berries, oranges), vegetables (spinach, kale), nuts, and seeds.
- Benefits: Reduce oxidative stress, support immune function, and promote overall health.

Fiber

- Description: Fiber is essential for digestive health and can help regulate blood sugar levels.
- Sources: Whole grains, fruits, vegetables, legumes, nuts, and seeds.
- Benefits: Promotes healthy digestion, helps maintain stable blood sugar levels, and supports heart health.

Probiotics

- Description: Probiotics are beneficial bacteria that support gut health and immune function.
- Sources: Yogurt, kefir, sauerkraut, kimchi, and other fermented foods.
- Benefits: Improve digestive health, enhance immune function, and may reduce inflammation.

Hydration

- Description: Adequate hydration is crucial for overall health and helps the body function optimally.
- Sources: Water, herbal teas, and hydrating fruits and vegetables (cucumbers, watermelon).
- Benefits: Maintains body temperature, supports digestion, and ensures proper circulation and nutrient transport.

Foods to Include in Your Diet

Lean Proteins
- Description: Proteins are essential for tissue repair, immune function, and maintaining muscle mass. Lean proteins offer these benefits without the excess fats that can contribute to other health issues.
- Examples:
  - Poultry: Chicken and turkey are excellent sources of lean protein.
  - Fish: Salmon, mackerel, and tuna provide protein and omega-3 fatty acids, which have anti-inflammatory properties.
  - Eggs: Rich in protein and essential vitamins.
  - Legumes: Beans, lentils, and chickpeas are great plant-based protein sources.
  - Low-fat dairy: Milk, yogurt, and cheese offer protein and calcium without excessive fat.
- Benefits: Supports muscle maintenance, boosts immune function, and aids in recovery.

Whole Grains
- Description: Whole grains are packed with fiber, vitamins, and minerals, providing sustained energy and supporting digestive health.
- Examples:
  - Brown Rice: A nutrient-dense alternative to white rice.
  - Quinoa: A complete protein source and rich in fiber.
  - Oats: Great for breakfast and high in soluble fiber.
  - Whole Wheat: Bread, pasta, and other whole wheat products.
  - Barley and Bulgur: Nutritious grains that can be used in various dishes.
- Benefits: Promotes healthy digestion, stabilizes blood sugar levels, and provides long-lasting energy.

Fruits
- Description: Fruits are rich in vitamins, minerals, antioxidants, and fiber. They play a crucial role in boosting the immune system and overall health.
- Examples:
  - Berries: Blueberries, strawberries, and raspberries are high in antioxidants.
  - Citrus Fruits: Oranges, lemons, and grapefruits provide vitamin C.
  - Apples and Pears: Good sources of fiber and various vitamins.
  - Bananas: Rich in potassium and easy to digest.
  - Kiwi and Papaya: Loaded with vitamins and digestive enzymes.
- Benefits: Enhances immune function, reduces inflammation, and improves digestion.

Vegetables

- Description: Vegetables are essential for their vitamins, minerals, fiber, and antioxidants. They support immune health and provide the nutrients necessary for overall well-being.
- Examples:
  - Leafy Greens: Spinach, kale, and Swiss chard are nutrient powerhouses.
  - Cruciferous Vegetables: Broccoli, cauliflower, and Brussels sprouts contain cancer-fighting compounds.
  - Root Vegetables: Carrots, sweet potatoes, and beets are rich in vitamins and minerals.
  - Bell Peppers: High in vitamin C and antioxidants.
  - Tomatoes: Packed with lycopene, a powerful antioxidant.
- Benefits: Boosts immune system, fights inflammation, and supports overall health.

Healthy Fats

- Description: Healthy fats are crucial for nutrient absorption, brain health, and reducing inflammation. They provide essential fatty acids that the body cannot produce on its own.
- Examples:
  - Avocados: Rich in monounsaturated fats and fiber.
  - Nuts and Seeds: Almonds, walnuts, chia seeds, and flaxseeds provide omega-3 fatty acids.
  - Olive Oil: A healthy fat for cooking and dressing salads.
  - Fatty Fish: Salmon, mackerel, and sardines are excellent sources of omega-3s.
  - Coconut Oil: Contains medium-chain triglycerides (MCTs) that are easily digested and used for energy.
- Benefits: Reduces inflammation, supports brain function, and improves heart health.

Probiotics and Fermented Foods

- Description: Probiotics and fermented foods support a healthy gut microbiome, which is crucial for immune function and digestion.
- Examples:
  - Yogurt: Contains live cultures that benefit gut health.
  - Kefir: A fermented milk drink rich in probiotics.
  - Sauerkraut and Kimchi: Fermented vegetables that provide beneficial bacteria.
  - Miso and Tempeh: Fermented soy products that add probiotics and protein.
  - Kombucha: A fermented tea rich in probiotics.
- Benefits: Improves digestion, boosts immune function, and enhances nutrient absorption.

Hydrating Foods

- Description: Staying hydrated is vital for overall health. Hydrating foods can help maintain fluid balance, especially important during treatment.
- Examples:
  - Cucumbers: High water content and low in calories.
  - Watermelon: Hydrating and rich in vitamins.
  - Citrus Fruits: Oranges, grapefruits, and lemons.
  - Tomatoes: High in water and nutrients.
  - Leafy Greens: Spinach and lettuce contain significant amounts of water.
- Benefits: Maintains hydration, supports kidney function, and helps regulate body temperature.

Spices and Herbs

- Description: Spices and herbs not only add flavor to dishes but also offer numerous health benefits due to their antioxidant and anti-inflammatory properties.
- Examples:
  - Turmeric: Contains curcumin, which has anti-inflammatory and antioxidant effects.
  - Ginger: Known for its anti-nausea and anti-inflammatory properties.
  - Garlic: Boosts the immune system and has antimicrobial properties.
  - Cinnamon: Helps regulate blood sugar levels.
  - Basil and Oregano: Rich in antioxidants and vitamins.
- Benefits: Enhances flavor, reduces inflammation, and supports overall health.

Foods to Avoid

Processed and Red Meats
- Description: Processed meats are those that have been preserved by smoking, curing, salting, or adding chemical preservatives. Red meats refer to beef, pork, lamb, and goat.
- Examples: Bacon, sausages, hot dogs, deli meats, beef, pork, lamb.
- **Reasons to Avoid:**
  - Carcinogenic Properties: Processed meats are classified as Group 1 carcinogens by the World Health Organization, meaning there is sufficient evidence that they cause cancer in humans. Red meats are classified as Group 2A, indicating they are probably carcinogenic.
  - Inflammation: High consumption of processed and red meats can increase inflammation in the body, which may negatively impact CLL management.
- Healthier Alternatives: Opt for lean proteins such as poultry, fish, legumes, and plant-based proteins.

High-Sugar Foods and Beverages
- Description: Foods and drinks high in added sugars can lead to various health issues, including obesity, diabetes, and cardiovascular disease.
- Examples: Sugary drinks (sodas, fruit juices with added sugar), candies, cakes, cookies, pastries, ice cream.
- **Reasons to Avoid:**
  - Blood Sugar Spikes: High-sugar foods can cause rapid increases in blood sugar levels, leading to insulin resistance and diabetes.
  - Weight Gain: Excessive sugar intake can contribute to weight gain, which may negatively impact overall health and treatment outcomes.
  - Immune Suppression: High sugar consumption can weaken the immune system, making it harder for the body to fight infections.
- Healthier Alternatives: Choose whole fruits, natural sweeteners like honey or maple syrup in moderation, and beverages like water, herbal teas, and unsweetened fruit juices.

Refined Carbohydrates
- Description: Refined carbohydrates are processed foods that have had most of their nutrients and fiber removed.
- Examples: White bread, white rice, pasta, pastries, and many packaged snack foods.

- **Reasons to Avoid:**
  - Nutrient Deficiency: Refined carbs lack essential nutrients and fiber, providing empty calories.
  - Blood Sugar Control: They can cause rapid spikes and drops in blood sugar levels, which can be detrimental to overall health.
  - Inflammation: High intake of refined carbohydrates is linked to increased inflammation in the body.
- Healthier Alternatives: Opt for whole grains like brown rice, quinoa, whole wheat bread, and whole grain pasta.

Trans Fats and Hydrogenated Oils

- Description: Trans fats are artificial fats created through hydrogenation, a process that solidifies liquid oils. These fats are found in many processed foods.
- Examples: Margarine, shortening, fried foods, baked goods (like cookies, cakes, and pies), and many packaged snacks.
- **Reasons to Avoid:**
  - Heart Health: Trans fats increase bad cholesterol (LDL) and decrease good cholesterol (HDL), raising the risk of heart disease.
  - Inflammation: They contribute to systemic inflammation, which can exacerbate health issues.
  - Cancer Risk: Some studies suggest a potential link between trans fats and increased cancer risk.
- Healthier Alternatives: Use healthy fats like olive oil, avocado oil, and coconut oil. Choose products labeled as trans fat-free.

Excessive Salt

- Description: High salt intake can lead to hypertension and other cardiovascular problems.
- Examples: Processed foods, canned soups, fast food, salty snacks (chips, pretzels), and certain condiments (soy sauce, ketchup).
- **Reasons to Avoid:**
  - Blood Pressure: Excessive salt can increase blood pressure, leading to cardiovascular issues.
  - Kidney Function: High salt intake can strain the kidneys and impair their function.
  - Fluid Retention: Salt can cause the body to retain water, leading to swelling and discomfort.
- Healthier Alternatives: Use herbs and spices to flavor food, choose low-sodium or sodium-free products, and cook fresh meals at home.

Alcohol
- Description: Alcohol can interfere with the body's ability to fight infections and may interact negatively with medications.
- Examples: Beer, wine, spirits, and cocktails.
- **Reasons to Avoid:**
  - Immune Function: Alcohol can suppress the immune system, making it harder to fend off infections.
  - Medication Interactions: It can interact with medications, reducing their effectiveness or causing harmful side effects.
  - Liver Health: Excessive alcohol consumption can damage the liver, which is crucial for detoxifying the body and metabolizing medications.
- Healthier Alternatives: Choose non-alcoholic beverages like sparkling water, herbal teas, and freshly squeezed juices.

Unpasteurized Products
- Description: Unpasteurized products may contain harmful bacteria that can cause infections, especially in individuals with compromised immune systems.
- Examples: Raw milk, certain cheeses (like feta, brie, and blue cheese), and unpasteurized juices or ciders.
- **Reasons to Avoid:**
  - Infection Risk: Unpasteurized products can harbor bacteria such as E. coli, Salmonella, and Listeria, posing a serious risk of infection.
- Healthier Alternatives: Choose pasteurized dairy products and juices, which have been treated to kill harmful bacteria.

Foods High in Saturated Fats
- Description: Saturated fats are typically solid at room temperature and are found in animal products and certain plant oils.
- Examples: Fatty cuts of meat, butter, lard, full-fat dairy products, and coconut oil.
- **Reasons to Avoid:**
  - Heart Health: High intake of saturated fats can raise cholesterol levels and increase the risk of heart disease.
  - Inflammation: Saturated fats can contribute to systemic inflammation, which may worsen CLL symptoms.
- Healthier Alternatives: Opt for sources of healthy fats like olive oil, avocado, nuts, and seeds.

Artificial Sweeteners and Additives

- Description: Artificial sweeteners and additives are often found in processed foods and beverages, offering little nutritional value.
- Examples: Aspartame, sucralose, saccharin, and food colorings.
- **Reasons to Avoid:**
  - Digestive Issues: Some artificial sweeteners can cause bloating, gas, and other digestive problems.
  - Health Concerns: Long-term effects of many artificial additives are still not fully understood, and some studies suggest potential health risks.
- Healthier Alternatives: Use natural sweeteners like honey or maple syrup in moderation, and choose whole, unprocessed foods.

The Importance of Hydration for CLL Patients

Why Hydration Matters
Hydration is essential for maintaining the body's normal physiological functions. Water makes up about 60% of the human body and is crucial for:

1. **Cell Function and Structure**
   - Water is a key component of cells and is involved in maintaining their structure and function. Proper hydration ensures that cells can operate efficiently, supporting overall health.
2. **Nutrient Transportation**
   - Hydration aids in the transport of nutrients and oxygen to cells, ensuring that the body gets the necessary components for energy production and repair processes.
3. **Waste Removal**
   - Adequate water intake helps the kidneys filter waste products from the blood and excrete them through urine. This detoxification process is vital for preventing the buildup of harmful substances in the body.
4. Temperature Regulation
   - Water helps regulate body temperature through sweating and respiration. This is particularly important for maintaining homeostasis and preventing overheating.
5. **Joint Lubrication**
   - Water acts as a lubricant for joints, reducing friction and allowing for smooth movement. This can help prevent joint pain and stiffness.

Specific Benefits for CLL Patients
For individuals with CLL, hydration plays an even more critical role due to the disease and its treatments:

1. **Managing Treatment Side Effects**
   - Chemotherapy and Hydration: Many CLL patients undergo chemotherapy, which can cause dehydration through side effects like nausea, vomiting, and diarrhea. Drinking enough water helps mitigate these effects, maintaining hydration and supporting the body's ability to recover.
   - Medication Metabolism: Proper hydration aids in the metabolism and clearance of medications, ensuring they work effectively and reducing the risk of toxicity.
2. **Supporting the Immune System**
   - Hydration is crucial for maintaining a robust immune system. Adequate fluid intake ensures that the lymphatic system, a key component of the immune system, can function properly. This helps the body fight infections and manage the disease more effectively.

3. Improving Energy Levels

- Fatigue is a common symptom of CLL. Staying well-hydrated can help improve energy levels and combat fatigue, making it easier for patients to engage in daily activities and maintain a better quality of life.

4. Promoting Digestive Health

- Hydration supports digestive health by aiding in the breakdown and absorption of nutrients. It also helps prevent constipation, a common issue for individuals undergoing cancer treatment.

5. Enhancing Skin Health

- Dehydration can lead to dry and flaky skin. Adequate water intake helps maintain skin hydration, improving its appearance and reducing the risk of skin infections.

6. Mental Clarity and Mood

- Proper hydration is essential for brain function. Dehydration can lead to confusion, irritability, and difficulty concentrating. Staying hydrated can help maintain mental clarity and improve mood.

Signs of Dehydration

Recognizing the signs of dehydration is crucial for timely intervention. Symptoms include:

- Thirst: A primary indicator that the body needs more fluids.
- Dry Mouth and Skin: Lack of moisture in the mouth and skin.
- Dark-Colored Urine: Indicates concentrated urine, a sign of inadequate fluid intake.
- Fatigue: Feeling unusually tired or lethargic.
- Dizziness: Lightheadedness or feeling faint.
- Headaches: Persistent headaches can be a sign of dehydration.
- Decreased Urination: Less frequent urination is a sign of reduced fluid intake.

Practical Tips for Maintaining Hydration

Maintaining proper hydration involves more than just drinking water. Here are practical tips to help CLL patients stay hydrated:

1. Set Hydration Goals
   - Aim to drink at least 8-10 glasses of water daily, but individual needs may vary based on body weight, activity level, and specific health conditions. Consult with a healthcare provider for personalized recommendations.
2. Monitor Fluid Intake
   - Keep track of daily fluid intake using a journal or a smartphone app. This can help ensure that hydration goals are met consistently.
3. Incorporate Hydrating Foods
   - Include foods with high water content in the diet. Examples include cucumbers, watermelon, oranges, strawberries, and leafy greens. Soups and broths are also excellent sources of hydration.

4. Create a Hydration Routine

- Establish a routine by drinking water at specific times of the day, such as upon waking, before meals, and before bedtime. Consistent habits can help maintain hydration levels.

5. Flavor Water Naturally

- Enhance the taste of water by adding natural flavorings like lemon, lime, cucumber slices, or mint leaves. This can make drinking water more enjoyable.

6. Carry a Water Bottle

- Keep a reusable water bottle handy throughout the day. This makes it easy to sip water regularly, especially when on the go.

7. Avoid Dehydrating Beverages

- Limit the intake of caffeinated and alcoholic beverages, as they can lead to dehydration. If consumed, balance them with additional water intake.

8. Use Hydration Reminders

- Set reminders on a phone or use hydration reminder apps to prompt regular drinking throughout the day.

9. Monitor Urine Color

- Use urine color as an indicator of hydration status. Light yellow or clear urine typically indicates adequate hydration.

10. Adjust for Activity and Environment

- Increase fluid intake during hot weather, physical activity, or when experiencing fever or illness to compensate for additional fluid loss.

Breakfast Recipes

1. Oatmeal with Fresh Berries
Servings: 2
Cooking Time: 10 minutes
Ingredients:
- 1 cup rolled oats
- 2 cups water or unsweetened almond milk
- 1/2 teaspoon ground cinnamon
- 1 cup mixed fresh berries (blueberries, strawberries, raspberries)
- 1 tablespoon chia seeds
- 1 tablespoon honey or maple syrup
- 1/4 cup chopped nuts (almonds, walnuts)

Instructions:
1. In a medium saucepan, bring the water or almond milk to a boil.
2. Stir in the oats and reduce the heat to low. Cook, stirring occasionally, for about 5 minutes or until the oats are tender and the liquid is absorbed.
3. Add the ground cinnamon and stir to combine.
4. Divide the oatmeal into two bowls.
5. Top each bowl with mixed fresh berries, chia seeds, chopped nuts, and a drizzle of honey or maple syrup.

Nutritional Information (per serving):
- Calories: 300
- Protein: 8g
- Carbohydrates: 48g
- Dietary Fiber: 9g
- Sugars: 15g
- Fat: 11g
- Saturated Fat: 1g
- Sodium: 10mg

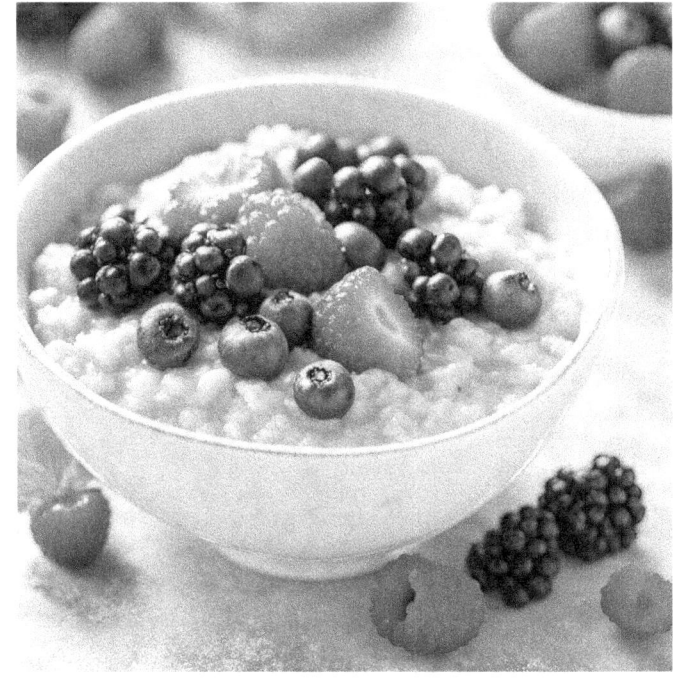

2. Greek Yogurt with Honey and Nuts

Servings: 1
Cooking Time: 5 minutes
Ingredients:

- 1 cup plain Greek yogurt
- 1 tablespoon honey
- 1/4 cup mixed nuts (almonds, walnuts, pistachios), chopped
- 1 tablespoon chia seeds
- 1/2 cup fresh fruit (berries or sliced banana)

Instructions:

1. Spoon the Greek yogurt into a serving bowl.
2. Drizzle the honey over the yogurt.
3. Sprinkle the chopped nuts, chia seeds, and fresh fruit on top.
4. Serve immediately.

Nutritional Information (per serving):

- Calories: 350
- Protein: 20g
- Carbohydrates: 30g
- Dietary Fiber: 5g
- Sugars: 20g
- Fat: 18g
- Saturated Fat: 3g
- Sodium: 60mg

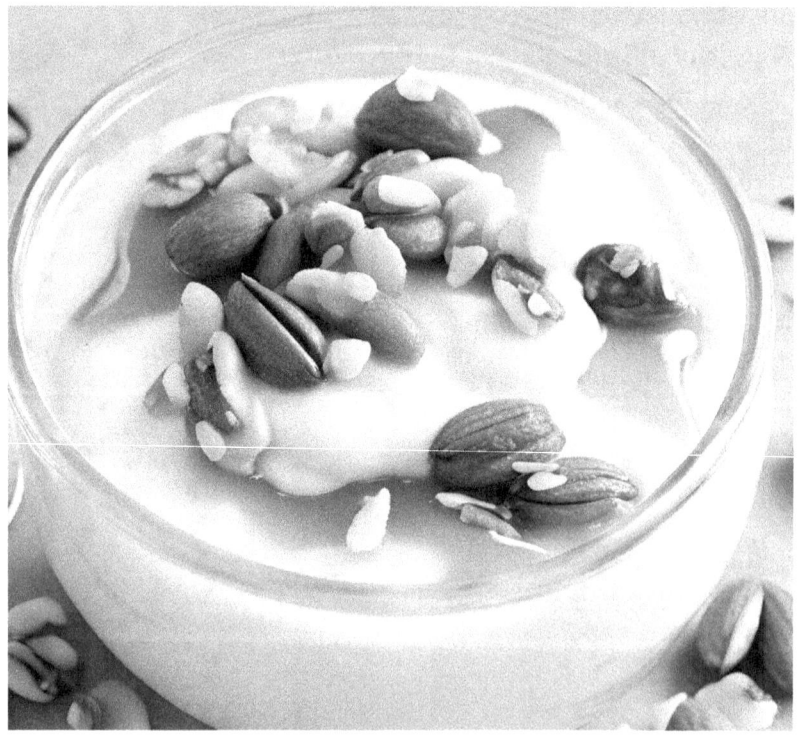

3. Green Smoothie

Servings: 2
Cooking Time: 5 minutes
Ingredients:

- 2 cups fresh spinach
- 1 banana
- 1 cup unsweetened almond milk
- 1/2 cup plain Greek yogurt
- 1 tablespoon chia seeds
- 1 tablespoon honey or maple syrup
- 1/2 cup ice cubes

Instructions:

1. Place all the ingredients in a blender.
2. Blend until smooth and creamy.
3. Pour into two glasses and serve immediately.

Nutritional Information (per serving):

- Calories: 200
- Protein: 8g
- Carbohydrates: 33g
- Dietary Fiber: 5g
- Sugars: 19g
- Fat: 5g
- Saturated Fat: 1g
- Sodium: 80mg

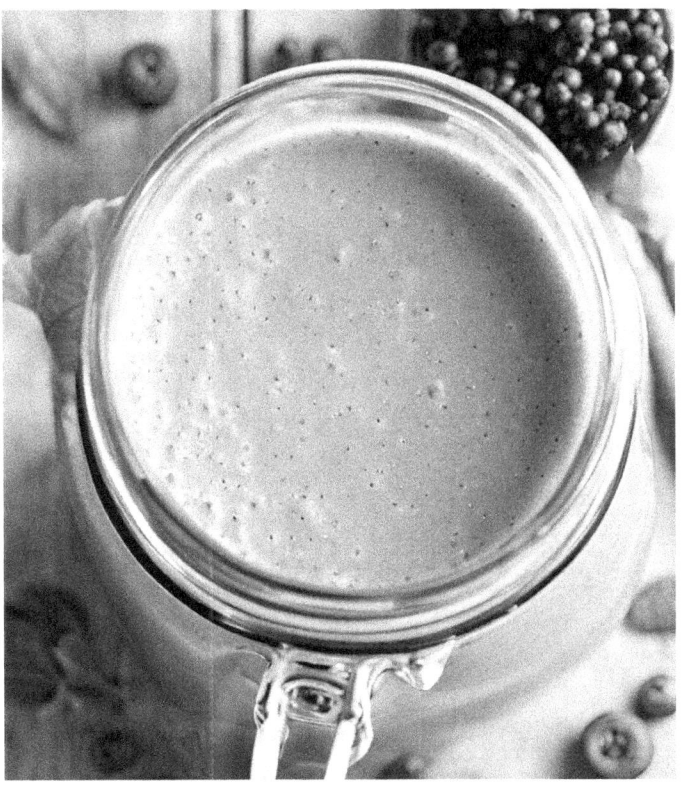

4. Quinoa Breakfast Bowl
Servings: 2
Cooking Time: 20 minutes
Ingredients:

- 1/2 cup quinoa, rinsed
- 1 cup water
- 1/2 teaspoon ground cinnamon
- 1/4 teaspoon vanilla extract
- 1 tablespoon honey or maple syrup
- 1/4 cup chopped nuts (almonds, walnuts)
- 1/2 cup fresh berries (blueberries, strawberries, raspberries)
- 1/4 cup unsweetened almond milk (optional)

Instructions:

1. In a medium saucepan, bring the quinoa and water to a boil.
2. Reduce the heat to low, cover, and simmer for about 15 minutes, or until the quinoa is cooked and the water is absorbed.
3. Stir in the ground cinnamon, vanilla extract, and honey or maple syrup.
4. Divide the quinoa into two bowls.
5. Top each bowl with chopped nuts, fresh berries, and a splash of almond milk if desired.

Nutritional Information (per serving):

- Calories: 280
- Protein: 8g
- Carbohydrates: 42g
- Dietary Fiber: 6g
- Sugars: 12g
- Fat: 10g
- Saturated Fat: 1g
- Sodium: 10mg

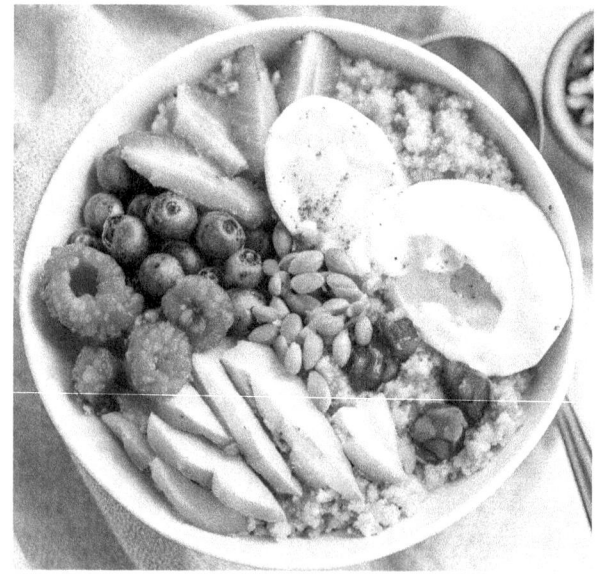

5. Egg White Omelet

Servings: 1
Cooking Time: 10 minutes
Ingredients:

- 4 egg whites
- 1/4 cup chopped spinach
- 1/4 cup diced tomatoes
- 1/4 cup diced bell peppers
- 1 tablespoon olive oil
- 1/4 cup feta cheese (optional)

Instructions:

1. Heat the olive oil in a non-stick skillet over medium heat.
2. Add the chopped spinach, tomatoes, and bell peppers. Sauté for 2-3 minutes until the vegetables are tender.
3. In a bowl, whisk the egg whites until slightly frothy.
4. Pour the egg whites into the skillet, spreading them evenly over the vegetables.
5. Cook until the eggs are set, about 3-4 minutes.
6. Sprinkle the feta cheese on top (if using) and fold the omelet in half.
7. Serve immediately.

Nutritional Information (per serving):

- Calories: 150
- Protein: 18g
- Carbohydrates: 5g
- Dietary Fiber: 1g
- Sugars: 2g
- Fat: 7g
- Saturated Fat: 2g
- Sodium: 220mg

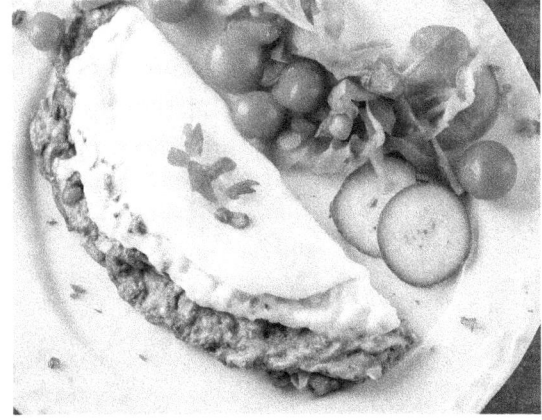

6. Whole Grain Pancakes
Servings: 4
Cooking Time: 20 minutes
Ingredients:

- 1 cup whole wheat flour
- 1 tablespoon baking powder
- 1/2 teaspoon ground cinnamon
- 1 cup unsweetened almond milk
- 1 large egg
- 1 tablespoon honey or maple syrup
- 1 teaspoon vanilla extract
- 1/4 cup blueberries (optional)
- Olive oil spray (for cooking)

Instructions:

1. In a large bowl, mix the whole wheat flour, baking powder, and ground cinnamon.
2. In another bowl, whisk together the almond milk, egg, honey or maple syrup, and vanilla extract.
3. Pour the wet ingredients into the dry ingredients and stir until just combined. Do not overmix.
4. Gently fold in the blueberries if using.
5. Heat a non-stick skillet or griddle over medium heat and lightly spray with olive oil.
6. Pour 1/4 cup of batter onto the skillet for each pancake. Cook until bubbles form on the surface, then flip and cook for another 1-2 minutes until golden brown.
7. Serve the pancakes warm with additional honey or maple syrup if desired.

Nutritional Information (per serving):

- Calories: 180
- Protein: 6g
- Carbohydrates: 29g
- Dietary Fiber: 4g
- Sugars: 7g
- Fat: 5g
- Saturated Fat: 1g
- Sodium: 200mg

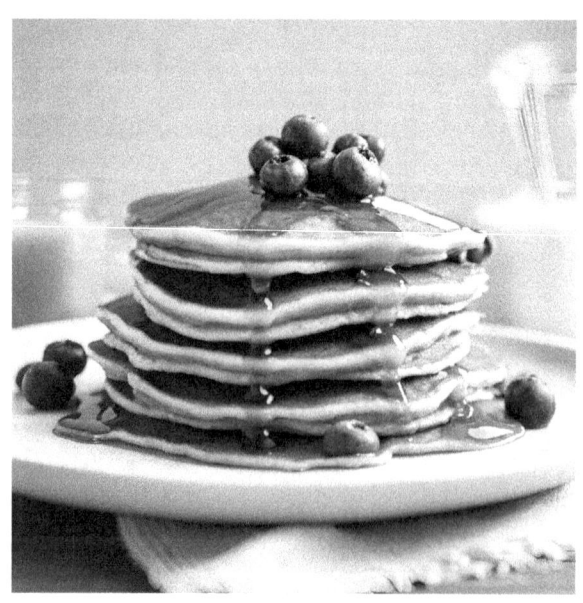

7. Overnight Oats

Servings: 2
Cooking Time: 5 minutes (plus overnight refrigeration)
Ingredients:

- 1 cup rolled oats
- 1 cup unsweetened almond milk
- 1/2 cup plain Greek yogurt
- 1 tablespoon chia seeds
- 1 tablespoon honey or maple syrup
- 1 teaspoon vanilla extract
- 1/2 cup fresh berries (blueberries, strawberries, raspberries)

Instructions:

1. In a medium bowl, combine the rolled oats, almond milk, Greek yogurt, chia seeds, honey or maple syrup, and vanilla extract.
2. Stir well to combine.
3. Divide the mixture into two jars or containers with lids.
4. Top each with fresh berries.
5. Cover and refrigerate overnight.
6. In the morning, stir and enjoy.

Nutritional Information (per serving):

- Calories: 280
- Protein: 10g
- Carbohydrates: 45g
- Dietary Fiber: 8g
- Sugars: 15g
- Fat: 7g
- Saturated Fat: 1g
- Sodium: 70mg

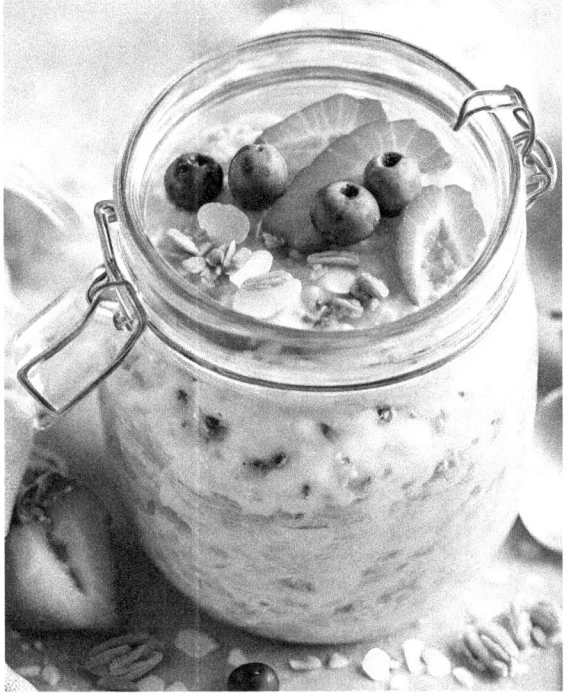

8. Smoothie Bowl
Servings: 1
Cooking Time: 10 minutes
Ingredients:

- 1 frozen banana
- 1/2 cup frozen berries
- 1/2 cup unsweetened almond milk
- 1/4 cup plain Greek yogurt
- 1 tablespoon chia seeds
- 1 tablespoon honey or maple syrup
- 1/4 cup granola (without added sugars)
- Fresh berries for topping
- Sliced almonds for topping

Instructions:

1. In a blender, combine the frozen banana, frozen berries, almond milk, Greek yogurt, chia seeds, and honey or maple syrup.
2. Blend until smooth and thick.
3. Pour into a bowl.
4. Top with granola, fresh berries, and sliced almonds.
5. Serve immediately.

Nutritional Information (per serving):

- Calories: 350
- Protein: 12g
- Carbohydrates: 60g
- Dietary Fiber: 9g
- Sugars: 25g
- Fat: 10g
- Saturated Fat: 1.5g
- Sodium: 90mg

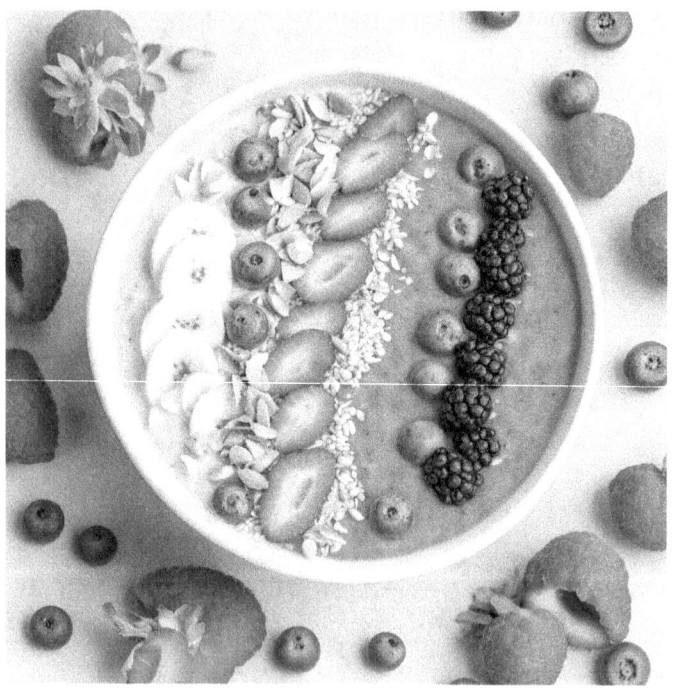

9. Buckwheat Porridge

Servings: 2
Cooking Time: 20 minutes
Ingredients:

- 1 cup buckwheat groats
- 2 cups water
- 1/2 teaspoon ground cinnamon
- 1 tablespoon honey or maple syrup
- 1/4 cup chopped nuts (almonds, walnuts)
- 1/2 cup fresh berries (blueberries, strawberries, raspberries)

Instructions:

1. Rinse the buckwheat groats under cold water.
2. In a medium saucepan, bring the water to a boil.
3. Add the buckwheat groats and reduce the heat to low. Simmer for about 15 minutes, or until the groats are tender and the water is absorbed.
4. Stir in the ground cinnamon and honey or maple syrup.
5. Divide the porridge into two bowls.
6. Top with chopped nuts and fresh berries.
7. Serve warm.

Nutritional Information (per serving):

- Calories: 300
- Protein: 8g
- Carbohydrates: 50g
- Dietary Fiber: 7g
- Sugars: 10g
- Fat: 10g
- Saturated Fat: 1g
- Sodium: 10mg

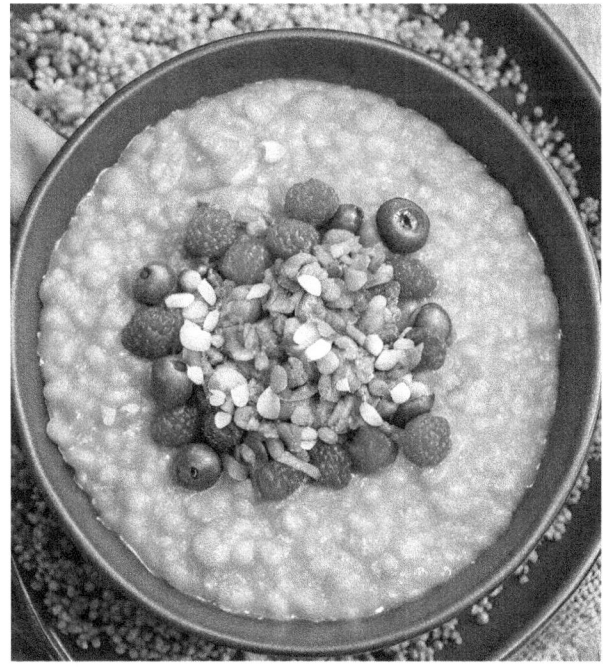

10. Nut Butter and Banana on Whole Grain Bread

Servings: 1
Cooking Time: 5 minutes
Ingredients:

- 2 slices whole grain bread
- 2 tablespoons natural almond or peanut butter
- 1 banana, sliced
- 1 teaspoon chia seeds

Instructions:

1. Toast the whole grain bread slices.
2. Spread the almond or peanut butter evenly on each slice.
3. Arrange the banana slices on top of the nut butter.
4. Sprinkle with chia seeds.
5. Serve immediately.

Nutritional Information (per serving):

- Calories: 350
- Protein: 10g
- Carbohydrates: 50g
- Dietary Fiber: 8g
- Sugars: 15g
- Fat: 15g
- Saturated Fat: 2g
- Sodium: 150mg

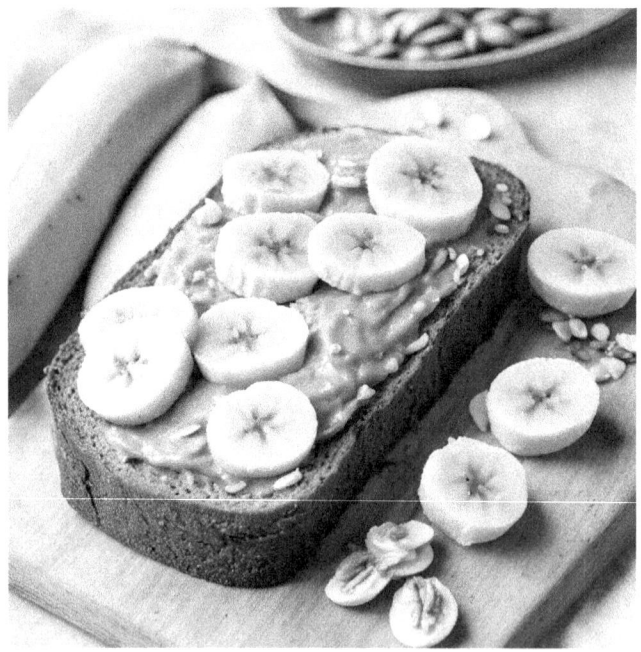

11. Apple Cinnamon Quinoa
Servings: 2
Cooking Time: 20 minutes
Ingredients:
- 1/2 cup quinoa, rinsed
- 1 cup water
- 1 apple, diced
- 1/2 teaspoon ground cinnamon
- 1 tablespoon honey or maple syrup
- 1/4 cup chopped walnuts
- 1/2 cup unsweetened almond milk

Instructions:
1. In a medium saucepan, bring the quinoa and water to a boil.
2. Reduce the heat to low, cover, and simmer for about 15 minutes, or until the quinoa is cooked and the water is absorbed.
3. Stir in the diced apple, ground cinnamon, and honey or maple syrup.
4. Divide the quinoa into two bowls.
5. Top each bowl with chopped walnuts and a splash of almond milk.
6. Serve warm.

Nutritional Information (per serving):
- Calories: 300
- Protein: 8g
- Carbohydrates: 45g
- Dietary Fiber: 6g
- Sugars: 12g
- Fat: 10g
- Saturated Fat: 1g
- Sodium: 20mg

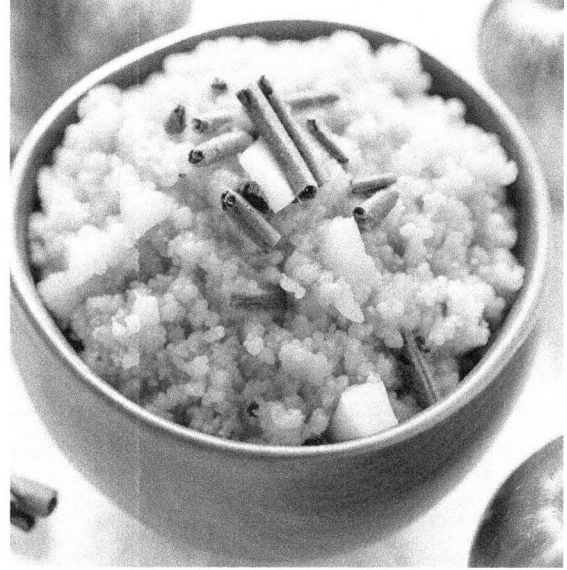

12. Berry Parfait

Servings: 2
Cooking Time: 10 minutes
Ingredients:

- 1 cup plain Greek yogurt
- 1 cup fresh berries (blueberries, strawberries, raspberries)
- 1/4 cup granola (without added sugars)
- 1 tablespoon honey or maple syrup
- 1 tablespoon chia seeds

Instructions:

1. In two serving glasses, layer the Greek yogurt, fresh berries, granola, and chia seeds.
2. Drizzle honey or maple syrup over the top.
3. Serve immediately.

Nutritional Information (per serving):

- Calories: 250
- Protein: 12g
- Carbohydrates: 40g
- Dietary Fiber: 6g
- Sugars: 18g
- Fat: 7g
- Saturated Fat: 1.5g
- Sodium: 80mg

13. Spinach and Feta Wrap

Servings: 1

Cooking Time: 10 minutes

Ingredients:

- 1 whole grain tortilla
- 1 cup fresh spinach leaves
- 1/4 cup crumbled feta cheese
- 1/4 cup diced tomatoes
- 1 tablespoon hummus

Instructions:

1. Warm the tortilla in a dry skillet over medium heat for about 1 minute.
2. Spread the hummus evenly over the tortilla.
3. Layer the spinach leaves, diced tomatoes, and crumbled feta cheese on top.
4. Roll up the tortilla tightly.
5. Serve immediately.

Nutritional Information (per serving):

- Calories: 250
- Protein: 10g
- Carbohydrates: 30g
- Dietary Fiber: 6g
- Sugars: 3g
- Fat: 10g
- Saturated Fat: 3g
- Sodium: 350mg

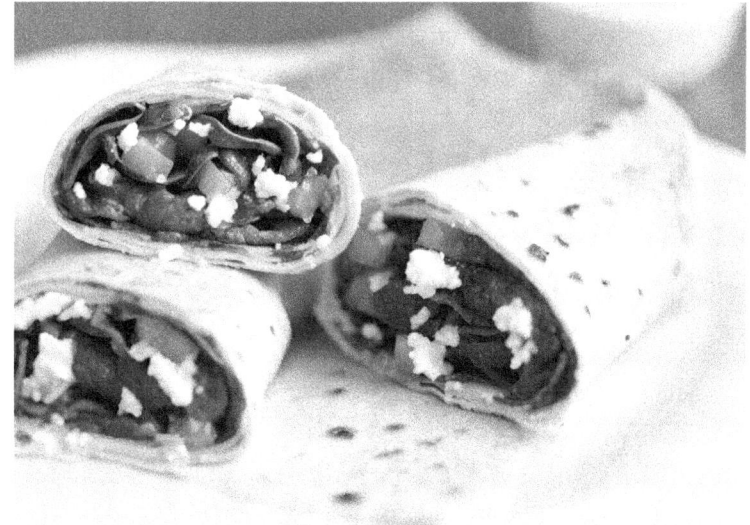

14. Zucchini Bread
Servings: 12 slices
Cooking Time: 1 hour
Ingredients:

- 1 1/2 cups whole wheat flour
- 1 teaspoon baking powder
- 1/2 teaspoon baking soda
- 1/2 teaspoon ground cinnamon
- 1/2 teaspoon ground nutmeg
- 2 large eggs
- 1/2 cup honey or maple syrup
- 1/2 cup unsweetened applesauce
- 1/4 cup olive oil
- 1 teaspoon vanilla extract
- 1 1/2 cups grated zucchini (about 1 medium zucchini)
- 1/2 cup chopped walnuts (optional)

Instructions:

1. Preheat the oven to 350°F (175°C). Grease a 9x5-inch loaf pan.
2. In a large bowl, whisk together the whole wheat flour, baking powder, baking soda, ground cinnamon, and ground nutmeg.
3. In another bowl, beat the eggs and mix in the honey or maple syrup, unsweetened applesauce, olive oil, and vanilla extract.
4. Add the wet ingredients to the dry ingredients and stir until just combined.
5. Fold in the grated zucchini and chopped walnuts, if using.
6. Pour the batter into the prepared loaf pan and smooth the top.
7. Bake for 45-50 minutes, or until a toothpick inserted into the center comes out clean.
8. Allow the bread to cool in the pan for 10 minutes before transferring it to a wire rack to cool completely.
9. Slice and serve.

Nutritional Information (per slice):

- Calories: 180
- Protein: 4g
- Carbohydrates: 25g
- Dietary Fiber: 3g
- Sugars: 12g
- Fat: 7g
- Saturated Fat: 1g
- Sodium: 90mg

15. Pumpkin Smoothie

Servings: 2
Cooking Time: 5 minutes
Ingredients:

- 1 cup canned pumpkin (unsweetened)
- 1 banana
- 1 cup unsweetened almond milk
- 1/2 cup plain Greek yogurt
- 1 tablespoon chia seeds
- 1 tablespoon honey or maple syrup
- 1/2 teaspoon ground cinnamon
- 1/4 teaspoon ground nutmeg
- 1/4 teaspoon ground ginger
- 1/2 cup ice cubes

Instructions:

1. Place all ingredients in a blender.
2. Blend until smooth and creamy.
3. Pour into two glasses and serve immediately.

Nutritional Information (per serving):

- Calories: 200
- Protein: 8g
- Carbohydrates: 38g
- Dietary Fiber: 7g
- Sugars: 20g
- Fat: 4g
- Saturated Fat: 1g
- Sodium: 90mg

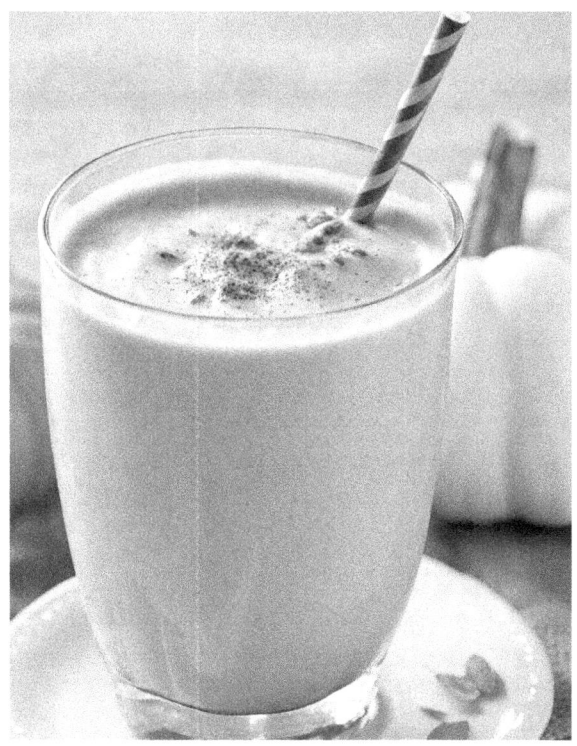

16. Pear and Walnut Salad
Servings: 2
Cooking Time: 10 minutes
Ingredients:
- 4 cups mixed greens (spinach, arugula, kale)
- 1 pear, thinly sliced
- 1/4 cup chopped walnuts
- 1/4 cup crumbled feta cheese (optional)
- 2 tablespoons balsamic vinaigrette

Instructions:
1. In a large bowl, combine the mixed greens, pear slices, walnuts, and feta cheese (if using).
2. Drizzle with balsamic vinaigrette.
3. Toss gently to combine.
4. Divide into two servings and serve immediately.

Nutritional Information (per serving):
- Calories: 200
- Protein: 5g
- Carbohydrates: 20g
- Dietary Fiber: 5g
- Sugars: 10g
- Fat: 12g
- Saturated Fat: 2g
- Sodium: 150mg

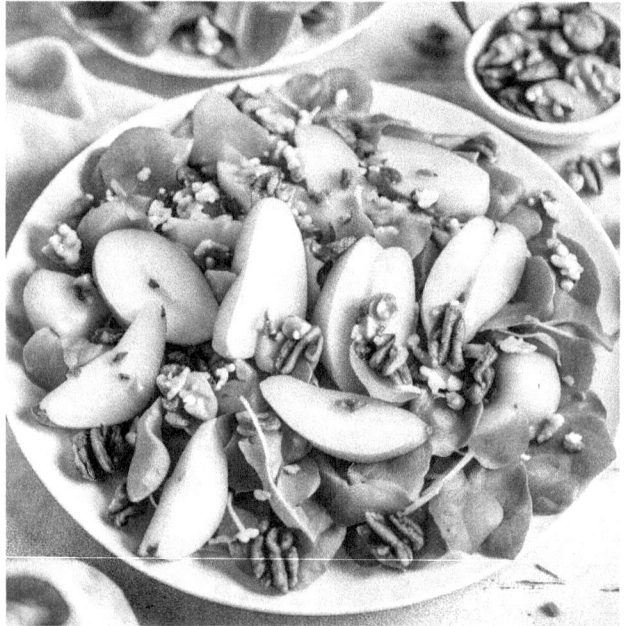

17. Berry Smoothie
Servings: 2
Cooking Time: 5 minutes
Ingredients:
- 1 cup mixed frozen berries (strawberries, blueberries, raspberries)
- 1 banana
- 1 cup unsweetened almond milk
- 1/2 cup plain Greek yogurt
- 1 tablespoon honey or maple syrup
- 1 tablespoon chia seeds
- 1/2 cup ice cubes

Instructions:
1. Place all ingredients in a blender.
2. Blend until smooth and creamy.
3. Pour into two glasses and serve immediately.

Nutritional Information (per serving):
- Calories: 220
- Protein: 9g
- Carbohydrates: 42g
- Dietary Fiber: 7g
- Sugars: 26g
- Fat: 4g
- Saturated Fat: 1g
- Sodium: 70mg

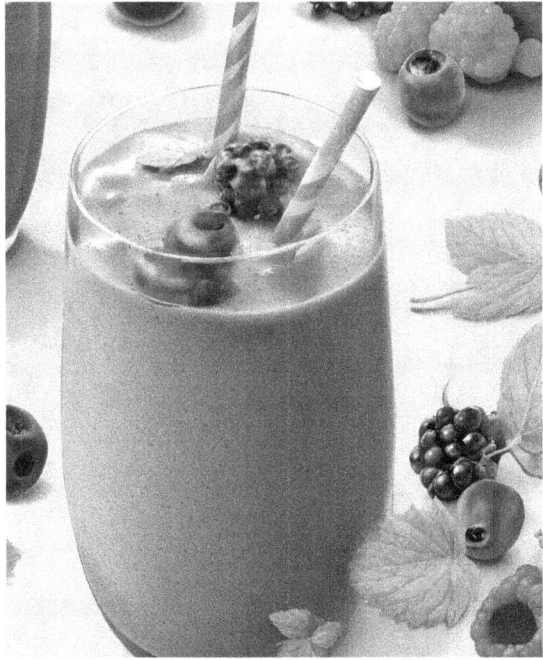

18. Granola and Yogurt Bowl

Servings: 1
Cooking Time: 5 minutes
Ingredients:

- 1 cup plain Greek yogurt
- 1/2 cup granola (without added sugars)
- 1/2 cup fresh berries (blueberries, strawberries, raspberries)
- 1 tablespoon chia seeds
- 1 tablespoon honey or maple syrup

Instructions:

1. Spoon the Greek yogurt into a serving bowl.
2. Top with granola, fresh berries, and chia seeds.
3. Drizzle with honey or maple syrup.
4. Serve immediately.

Nutritional Information (per serving):

- Calories: 350
- Protein: 20g
- Carbohydrates: 50g
- Dietary Fiber: 8g
- Sugars: 22g
- Fat: 10g
- Saturated Fat: 2g
- Sodium: 80mg

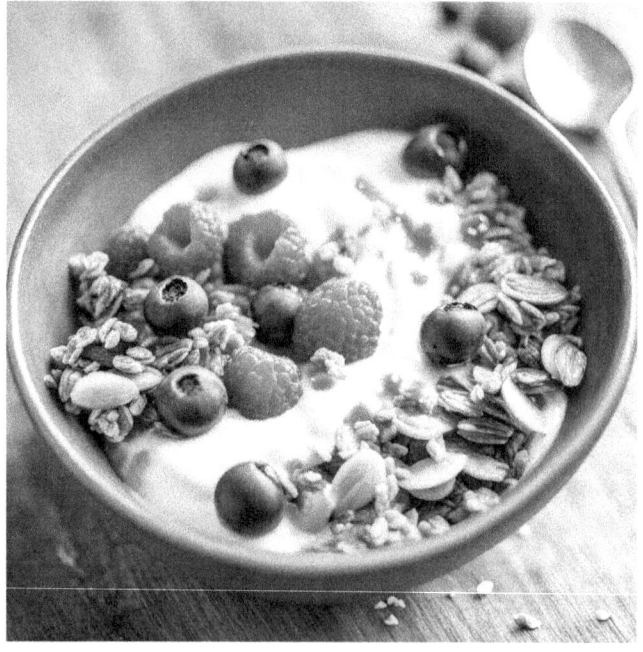

19. Banana Nut Muffins

Servings: 12 muffins
Cooking Time: 30 minutes
Ingredients:

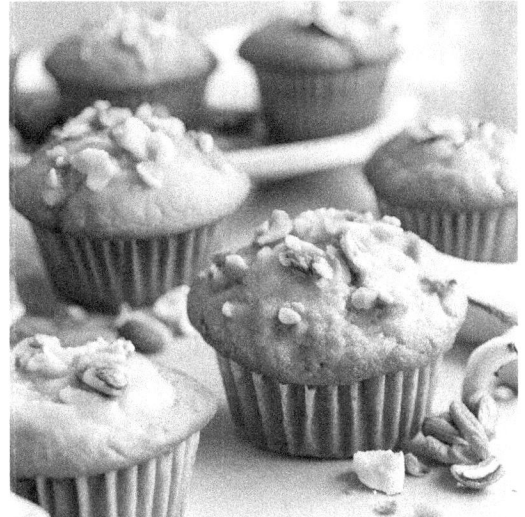

- 1 1/2 cups whole wheat flour
- 1 teaspoon baking soda
- 1/2 teaspoon ground cinnamon
- 1/4 teaspoon ground nutmeg
- 1/4 teaspoon ground ginger
- 1/4 cup olive oil
- 1/2 cup honey or maple syrup
- 2 large eggs
- 3 ripe bananas, mashed
- 1 teaspoon vanilla extract
- 1/2 cup chopped walnuts

Instructions:

1. Preheat the oven to 350°F (175°C). Line a muffin tin with paper liners or lightly grease it.
2. In a large bowl, whisk together the whole wheat flour, baking soda, ground cinnamon, ground nutmeg, and ground ginger.
3. In another bowl, mix the olive oil, honey or maple syrup, eggs, mashed bananas, and vanilla extract until well combined.
4. Add the wet ingredients to the dry ingredients and stir until just combined. Do not overmix.
5. Fold in the chopped walnuts.
6. Divide the batter evenly among the muffin cups.
7. Bake for 20-25 minutes, or until a toothpick inserted into the center comes out clean.
8. Allow the muffins to cool in the tin for 10 minutes before transferring them to a wire rack to cool completely.

Nutritional Information (per muffin):

- Calories: 180
- Protein: 4g
- Carbohydrates: 28g
- Dietary Fiber: 3g
- Sugars: 14g
- Fat: 7g
- Saturated Fat: 1g
- Sodium: 120mg

20. Blueberry Almond Overnight Oats
Servings: 2
Cooking Time: 5 minutes (plus overnight refrigeration)
Ingredients:
- 1 cup rolled oats
- 1 cup unsweetened almond milk
- 1/2 cup plain Greek yogurt
- 1 tablespoon chia seeds
- 1 tablespoon honey or maple syrup
- 1 teaspoon vanilla extract
- 1/2 cup fresh blueberries
- 1/4 cup sliced almonds

Instructions:
1. In a medium bowl, combine the rolled oats, almond milk, Greek yogurt, chia seeds, honey or maple syrup, and vanilla extract.
2. Stir well to combine.
3. Divide the mixture into two jars or containers with lids.
4. Top each with fresh blueberries and sliced almonds.
5. Cover and refrigerate overnight.
6. In the morning, stir and enjoy.

Nutritional Information (per serving):
- Calories: 310
- Protein: 11g
- Carbohydrates: 45g
- Dietary Fiber: 8g
- Sugars: 15g
- Fat: 10g
- Saturated Fat: 1g
- Sodium: 60mg

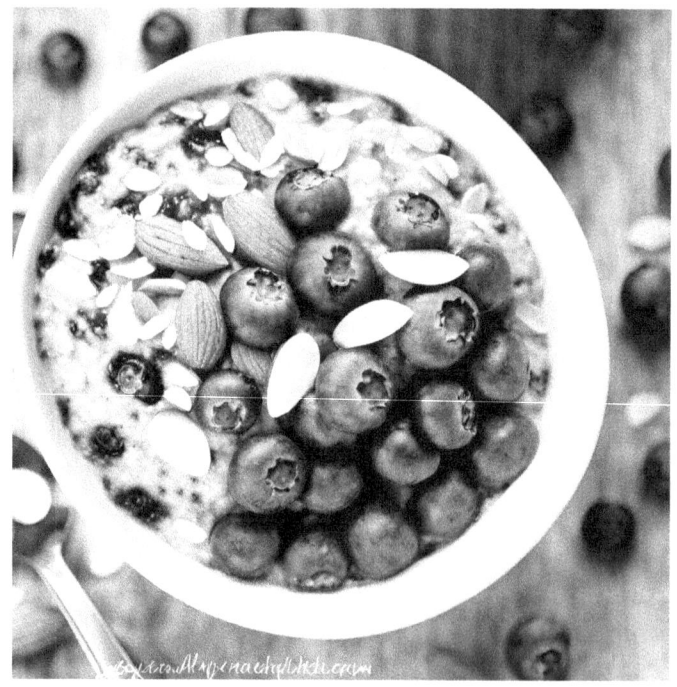

21. Hummus and Veggie Wrap

Servings: 1
Cooking Time: 10 minutes
Ingredients:

- 1 whole grain tortilla
- 3 tablespoons hummus
- 1/4 cup shredded carrots
- 1/4 cup cucumber slices
- 1/4 cup red bell pepper slices
- 1/4 cup baby spinach leaves
- 1 tablespoon chopped fresh parsley

Instructions:

1. Lay the whole grain tortilla flat on a clean surface.
2. Spread the hummus evenly over the tortilla.
3. Layer the shredded carrots, cucumber slices, red bell pepper slices, baby spinach leaves, and chopped parsley on top of the hummus.
4. Roll up the tortilla tightly.
5. Serve immediately or wrap in foil for an on-the-go meal.

Nutritional Information (per serving):

- Calories: 220
- Protein: 8g
- Carbohydrates: 30g
- Dietary Fiber: 8g
- Sugars: 4g
- Fat: 9g
- Saturated Fat: 1g
- Sodium: 350mg

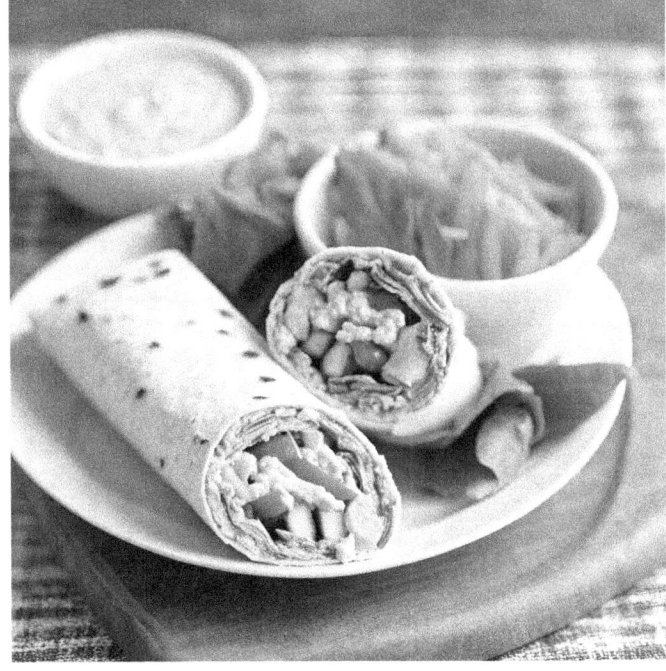

22. Pear and Almond Oatmeal
Servings: 2
Cooking Time: 10 minutes
Ingredients:
- 1 cup rolled oats
- 2 cups water or unsweetened almond milk
- 1 pear, diced
- 1/2 teaspoon ground cinnamon
- 1 tablespoon honey or maple syrup
- 1/4 cup sliced almonds

Instructions:
1. In a medium saucepan, bring the water or almond milk to a boil.
2. Stir in the rolled oats and reduce the heat to low. Cook, stirring occasionally, for about 5 minutes or until the oats are tender and the liquid is absorbed.
3. Add the diced pear, ground cinnamon, and honey or maple syrup. Stir to combine.
4. Divide the oatmeal into two bowls.
5. Top each bowl with sliced almonds.
6. Serve warm.

Nutritional Information (per serving):
- Calories: 300
- Protein: 7g
- Carbohydrates: 50g
- Dietary Fiber: 8g
- Sugars: 20g
- Fat: 8g
- Saturated Fat: 1g
- Sodium: 20mg

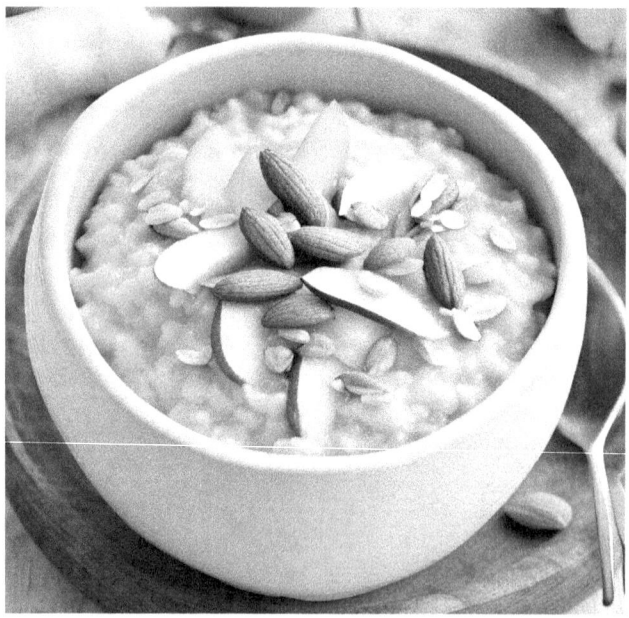

23. Carrot and Orange Smoothie
Servings: 2
Cooking Time: 5 minutes
Ingredients:

- 2 medium carrots, peeled and chopped
- 1 orange, peeled and segmented
- 1 banana
- 1 cup unsweetened almond milk
- 1/2 cup plain Greek yogurt
- 1 tablespoon honey or maple syrup
- 1/2 cup ice cubes

Instructions:

1. Place all ingredients in a blender.
2. Blend until smooth and creamy.
3. Pour into two glasses and serve immediately.

Nutritional Information (per serving):

- Calories: 200
- Protein: 6g
- Carbohydrates: 42g
- Dietary Fiber: 6g
- Sugars: 28g
- Fat: 3g
- Saturated Fat: 1g
- Sodium: 70mg

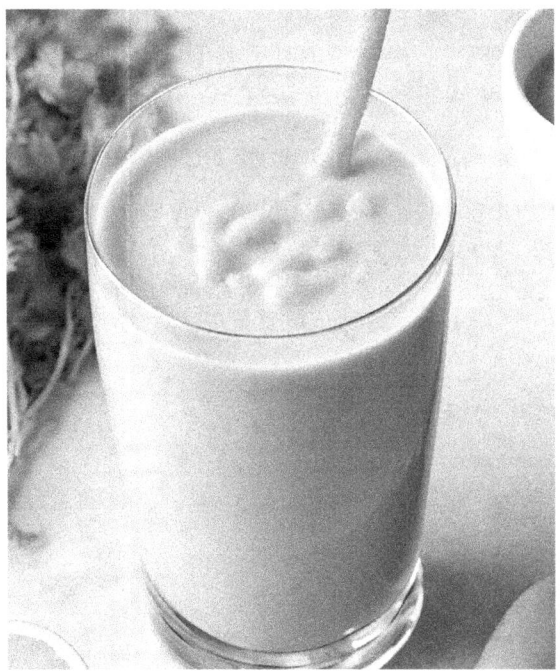

24. Almond Flour Pancakes

Servings: 4 (8 pancakes)
Cooking Time: 20 minutes
Ingredients:

- 2 cups almond flour
- 2 large eggs
- 1/4 cup unsweetened almond milk
- 1 tablespoon honey or maple syrup
- 1 teaspoon vanilla extract
- 1/2 teaspoon baking powder
- Olive oil spray (for cooking)

Instructions:

1. In a large bowl, whisk together the almond flour and baking powder.
2. In another bowl, beat the eggs and mix in the almond milk, honey or maple syrup, and vanilla extract.
3. Pour the wet ingredients into the dry ingredients and stir until just combined. Do not overmix.
4. Heat a non-stick skillet or griddle over medium heat and lightly spray with olive oil.
5. Pour 1/4 cup of batter onto the skillet for each pancake. Cook until bubbles form on the surface, then flip and cook for another 1-2 minutes until golden brown.
6. Serve the pancakes warm with additional honey or maple syrup if desired.

Nutritional Information (per serving):

- Calories: 250
- Protein: 10g
- Carbohydrates: 12g
- Dietary Fiber: 3g
- Sugars: 6g
- Fat: 20g
- Saturated Fat: 2g
- Sodium: 80mg

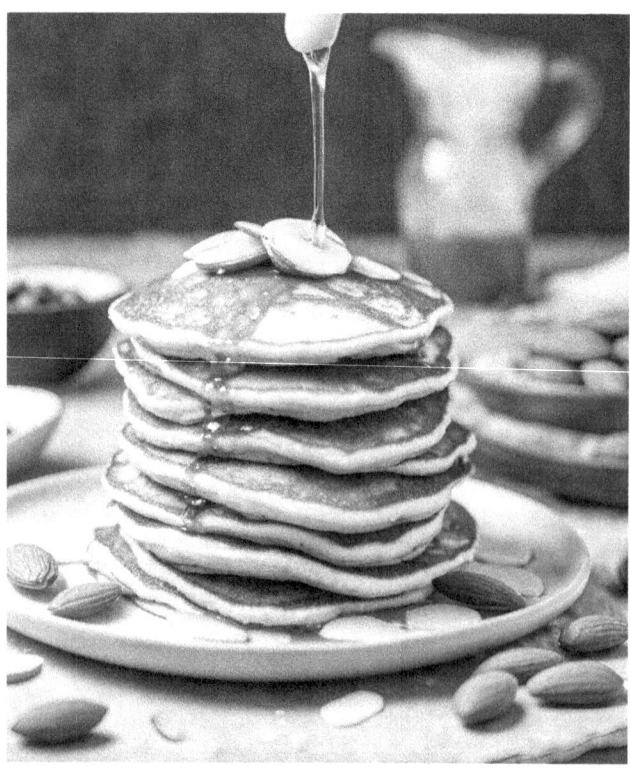

Fish & Seafood Recipes.

1. Grilled Salmon with Lemon and Dill
Servings: 4
Cooking Time: 20 minutes
Ingredients:

- 4 salmon fillets (about 6 ounces each)
- 2 tablespoons olive oil
- 2 tablespoons fresh lemon juice
- 2 tablespoons fresh dill, chopped
- 2 cloves garlic, minced
- 1 lemon, sliced into rounds

Instructions:

1. Preheat the grill to medium-high heat.
2. In a small bowl, mix the olive oil, lemon juice, dill, and garlic.
3. Brush the salmon fillets with the olive oil mixture on both sides.
4. Place the salmon fillets on the grill, skin-side down.
5. Grill for about 5-7 minutes on each side or until the salmon is cooked through and flakes easily with a fork.
6. Serve the salmon fillets with lemon slices on top.

Nutritional Information (per serving):

- Calories: 310
- Protein: 34g
- Carbohydrates: 2g
- Dietary Fiber: 0g
- Sugars: 0g
- Fat: 18g
- Saturated Fat: 3g
- Sodium: 60mg

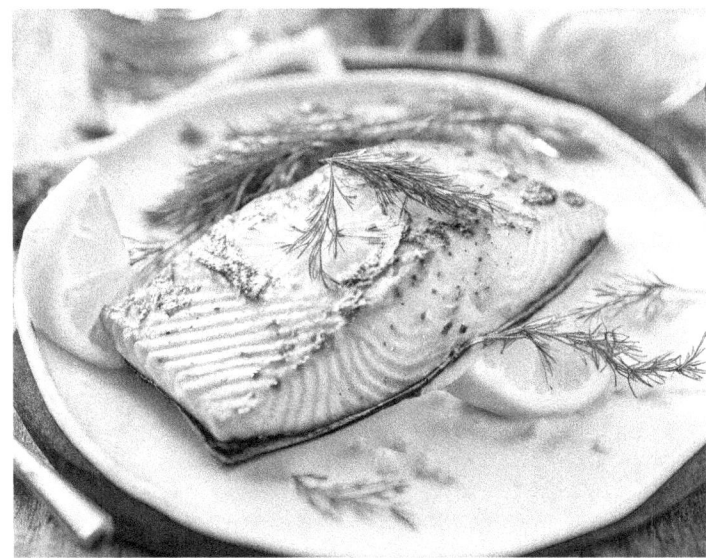

2. Baked Cod with Herbs
Servings: 4
Cooking Time: 25 minutes
Ingredients:

- 4 cod fillets (about 6 ounces each)
- 2 tablespoons olive oil
- 2 tablespoons fresh lemon juice
- 1 teaspoon dried oregano
- 1 teaspoon dried thyme
- 1 teaspoon dried basil
- 2 cloves garlic, minced
- 1 lemon, sliced into rounds

Instructions:

1. Preheat the oven to 375°F (190°C).
2. In a small bowl, mix the olive oil, lemon juice, oregano, thyme, basil, and garlic.
3. Place the cod fillets in a baking dish.
4. Brush the olive oil mixture over the cod fillets.
5. Arrange lemon slices on top of the fillets.
6. Bake for 15-20 minutes or until the cod is cooked through and flakes easily with a fork.
7. Serve immediately.

Nutritional Information (per serving):

- Calories: 220
- Protein: 32g
- Carbohydrates: 3g
- Dietary Fiber: 0g
- Sugars: 0g
- Fat: 9g
- Saturated Fat: 1.5g
- Sodium: 80mg

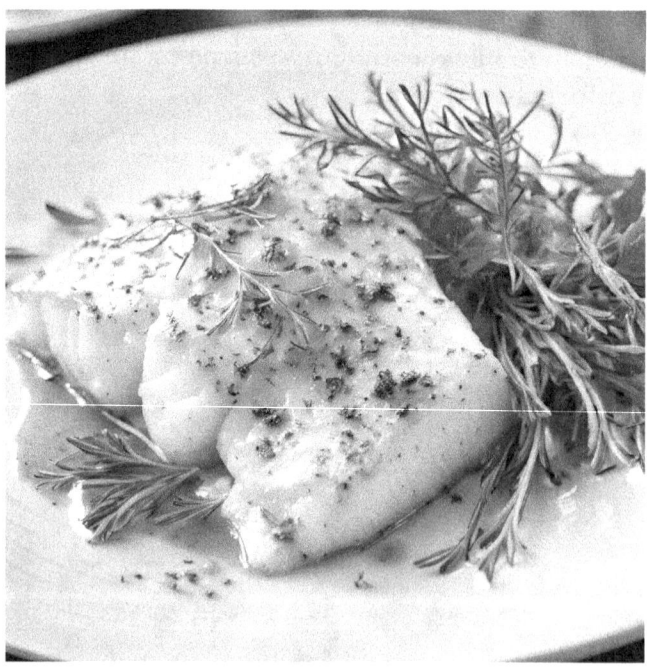

3. Steamed Tilapia with Ginger and Scallions
Servings: 4
Cooking Time: 20 minutes
Ingredients:
- 4 tilapia fillets (about 6 ounces each)
- 1 tablespoon fresh ginger, grated
- 2 cloves garlic, minced
- 4 scallions, sliced thinly
- 2 tablespoons soy sauce (low sodium)
- 2 tablespoons sesame oil

Instructions:
1. Prepare a steamer or set a steaming rack in a large pot with about 2 inches of water. Bring the water to a boil.
2. Place the tilapia fillets on a heatproof plate that fits inside the steamer.
3. Sprinkle the grated ginger, minced garlic, and sliced scallions over the tilapia.
4. Drizzle the soy sauce and sesame oil over the fillets.
5. Place the plate with the tilapia in the steamer. Cover and steam for about 10-12 minutes or until the fish is cooked through and flakes easily with a fork.
6. Serve immediately.

Nutritional Information (per serving):
- Calories: 220
- Protein: 32g
- Carbohydrates: 2g
- Dietary Fiber: 0g
- Sugars: 0g
- Fat: 9g
- Saturated Fat: 1.5g
- Sodium: 270mg

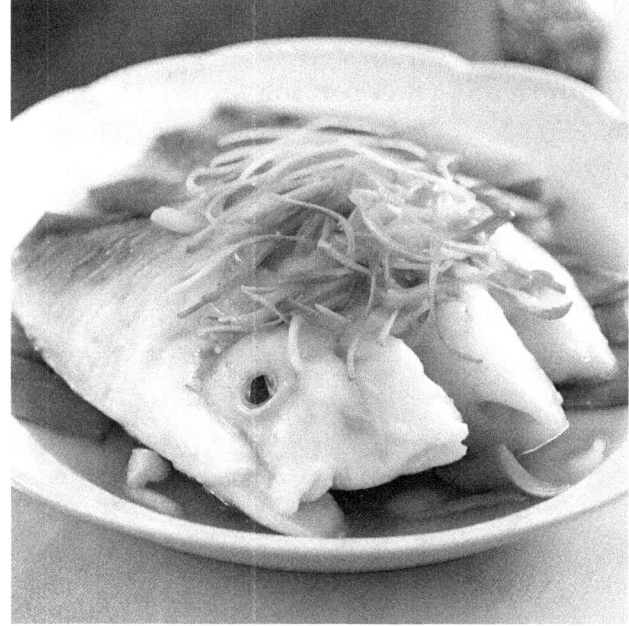

4. Shrimp Stir-Fry with Vegetables

Servings: 4

Cooking Time: 20 minutes

Ingredients:

- 1 pound shrimp, peeled and deveined
- 2 tablespoons olive oil
- 1 bell pepper, sliced
- 1 zucchini, sliced
- 1 carrot, julienned
- 2 cups broccoli florets
- 3 cloves garlic, minced
- 2 tablespoons soy sauce (low sodium)
- 1 tablespoon sesame oil
- 1 tablespoon fresh ginger, grated

Instructions:

1. Heat the olive oil in a large skillet or wok over medium-high heat.
2. Add the garlic and ginger, and sauté for about 1 minute until fragrant.
3. Add the bell pepper, zucchini, carrot, and broccoli to the skillet. Stir-fry for about 5-7 minutes until the vegetables are tender-crisp.
4. Add the shrimp to the skillet and cook for about 3-4 minutes until the shrimp turn pink and are cooked through.
5. Drizzle the soy sauce and sesame oil over the stir-fry and toss to combine.
6. Serve immediately.

Nutritional Information (per serving):

- Calories: 250
- Protein: 28g
- Carbohydrates: 10g
- Dietary Fiber: 3g
- Sugars: 4g
- Fat: 12g
- Saturated Fat: 2g
- Sodium: 500mg

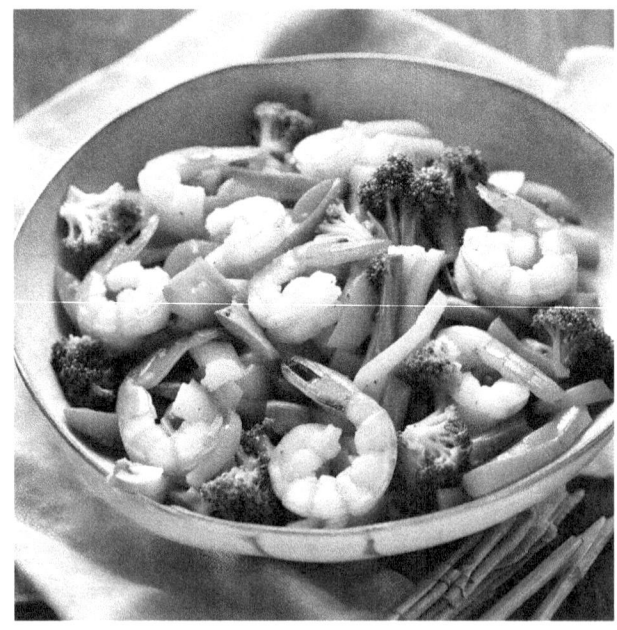

5. Tuna Salad with Avocado

Servings: 2

Cooking Time: 10 minutes

Ingredients:

- 2 cans tuna in water, drained
- 1 avocado, diced
- 1/4 cup red onion, finely chopped
- 1/4 cup celery, finely chopped
- 2 tablespoons plain Greek yogurt
- 1 tablespoon lemon juice
- 1 teaspoon Dijon mustard
- 1 tablespoon fresh parsley, chopped

Instructions:

1. In a medium bowl, combine the drained tuna, diced avocado, red onion, and celery.
2. In a small bowl, whisk together the Greek yogurt, lemon juice, and Dijon mustard.
3. Pour the dressing over the tuna mixture and gently toss to combine.
4. Garnish with chopped parsley.
5. Serve immediately.

Nutritional Information (per serving):

- Calories: 290
- Protein: 32g
- Carbohydrates: 10g
- Dietary Fiber: 6g
- Sugars: 2g
- Fat: 15g
- Saturated Fat: 2g
- Sodium: 350mg

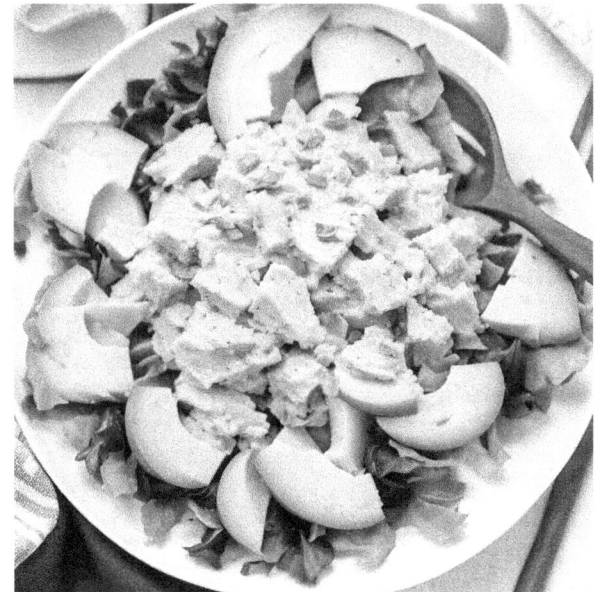

6. Salmon and Quinoa Bowl

Servings: 4
Cooking Time: 30 minutes
Ingredients:

- 1 cup quinoa, rinsed
- 2 cups water
- 4 salmon fillets (about 6 ounces each)
- 2 tablespoons olive oil
- 2 tablespoons fresh lemon juice
- 1 teaspoon dried oregano
- 1 avocado, sliced
- 1 cup cherry tomatoes, halved
- 1/2 cup red onion, thinly sliced
- 1/4 cup fresh parsley, chopped

Instructions:

1. In a medium saucepan, bring the water to a boil. Add the quinoa, reduce heat to low, cover, and simmer for 15 minutes or until the quinoa is cooked and the water is absorbed.
2. Preheat the oven to 375°F (190°C).
3. In a small bowl, mix the olive oil, lemon juice, and dried oregano.
4. Place the salmon fillets on a baking sheet lined with parchment paper. Brush the olive oil mixture over the salmon.
5. Bake the salmon for 15-20 minutes or until the salmon is cooked through and flakes easily with a fork.
6. Divide the cooked quinoa among four bowls.
7. Top each bowl with a salmon fillet, avocado slices, cherry tomatoes, red onion, and chopped parsley.
8. Serve immediately.

Nutritional Information (per serving):

- Calories: 450
- Protein: 35g
- Carbohydrates: 28g
- Dietary Fiber: 7g
- Sugars: 3g
- Fat: 22g
- Saturated Fat: 3g
- Sodium: 120mg

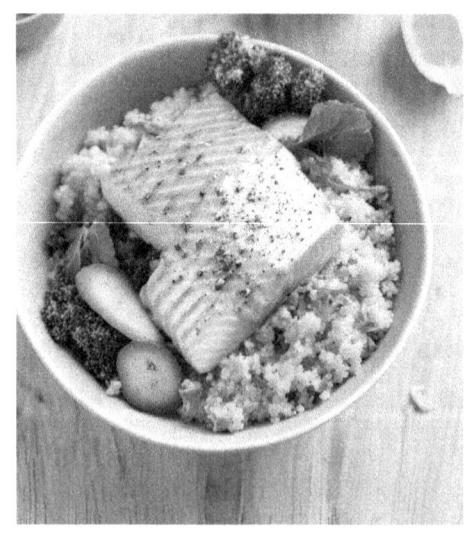

7. Baked Mackerel with Lemon
Servings: 4
Cooking Time: 25 minutes
Ingredients:
- 4 mackerel fillets (about 6 ounces each)
- 2 tablespoons olive oil
- 2 tablespoons fresh lemon juice
- 1 teaspoon dried thyme
- 2 cloves garlic, minced
- 1 lemon, sliced into rounds

Instructions:
1. Preheat the oven to 375°F (190°C).
2. In a small bowl, mix the olive oil, lemon juice, thyme, and minced garlic.
3. Place the mackerel fillets in a baking dish.
4. Brush the olive oil mixture over the mackerel fillets.
5. Arrange the lemon slices on top of the fillets.
6. Bake for 15-20 minutes, or until the mackerel is cooked through and flakes easily with a fork.
7. Serve immediately.

Nutritional Information (per serving):
- Calories: 300
- Protein: 30g
- Carbohydrates: 2g
- Dietary Fiber: 0g
- Sugars: 0g
- Fat: 20g
- Saturated Fat: 4g
- Sodium: 90mg

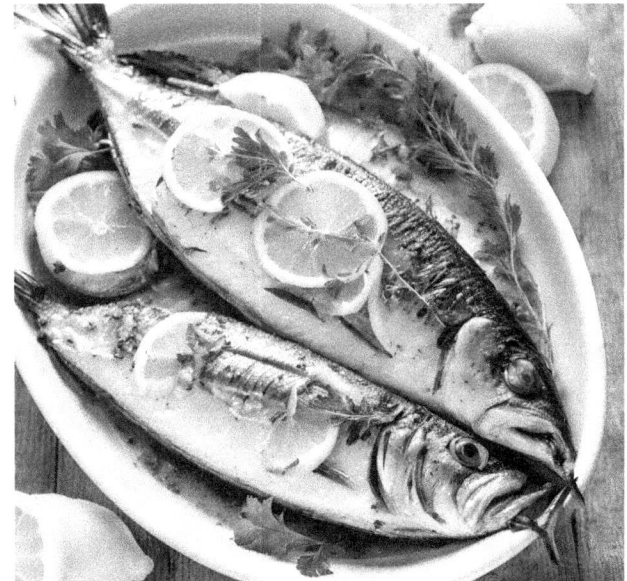

8. Fish Tacos

Servings: 4
Cooking Time: 20 minutes
Ingredients:

- 1 pound white fish fillets (such as cod or tilapia)
- 2 tablespoons olive oil
- 1 teaspoon cumin
- 1 teaspoon paprika
- 1 tablespoon lime juice
- 8 small corn tortillas
- 1 cup shredded red cabbage
- 1/2 cup diced tomatoes
- 1/4 cup chopped fresh cilantro
- 1 avocado, sliced
- Lime wedges, for serving

Instructions:

1. In a small bowl, mix the olive oil, cumin, paprika, and lime juice.
2. Brush the mixture over the fish fillets.
3. Heat a grill or skillet over medium-high heat.
4. Cook the fish for about 3-4 minutes on each side, or until cooked through and flaky.
5. Warm the corn tortillas in a dry skillet.
6. Assemble the tacos by placing the fish in the tortillas and topping with shredded cabbage, diced tomatoes, cilantro, and avocado slices.
7. Serve with lime wedges.

Nutritional Information (per serving):

- Calories: 310
- Protein: 25g
- Carbohydrates: 25g
- Dietary Fiber: 7g
- Sugars: 2g
- Fat: 15g
- Saturated Fat: 2g
- Sodium: 150mg

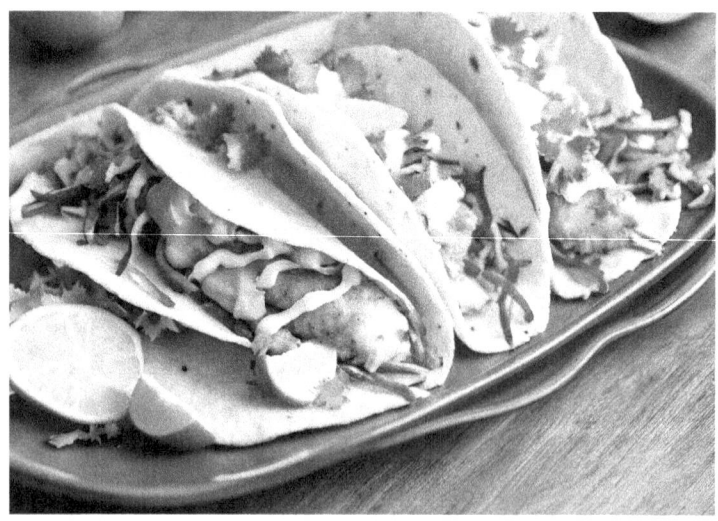

9. Lemon Garlic Tilapia

Servings: 4
Cooking Time: 20 minutes
Ingredients:

- 4 tilapia fillets (about 6 ounces each)
- 3 tablespoons olive oil
- 2 tablespoons fresh lemon juice
- 3 cloves garlic, minced
- 1 teaspoon dried oregano
- 1 lemon, sliced into rounds

Instructions:

1. Preheat the oven to 375°F (190°C).
2. In a small bowl, mix the olive oil, lemon juice, minced garlic, and oregano.
3. Place the tilapia fillets in a baking dish.
4. Brush the olive oil mixture over the tilapia fillets.
5. Arrange the lemon slices on top of the fillets.
6. Bake for 15 minutes, or until the tilapia is cooked through and flakes easily with a fork.
7. Serve immediately.

Nutritional Information (per serving):

- Calories: 220
- Protein: 30g
- Carbohydrates: 2g
- Dietary Fiber: 0g
- Sugars: 0g
- Fat: 10g
- Saturated Fat: 1.5g
- Sodium: 80mg

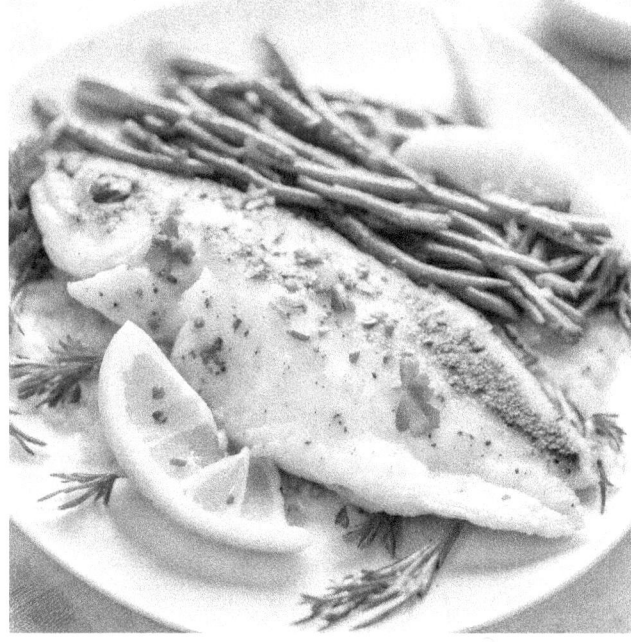

10. Broiled Salmon with Asparagus
Servings: 4
Cooking Time: 20 minutes
Ingredients:

- 4 salmon fillets (about 6 ounces each)
- 1 pound asparagus, trimmed
- 3 tablespoons olive oil
- 2 tablespoons fresh lemon juice
- 1 teaspoon dried dill
- 2 cloves garlic, minced

Instructions:

1. Preheat the broiler.
2. In a small bowl, mix 2 tablespoons of olive oil, lemon juice, dill, and minced garlic.
3. Place the salmon fillets on a baking sheet lined with foil.
4. Brush the olive oil mixture over the salmon fillets.
5. Toss the asparagus with the remaining tablespoon of olive oil and place next to the salmon on the baking sheet.
6. Broil for about 10-12 minutes, or until the salmon is cooked through and the asparagus is tender.
7. Serve immediately.

Nutritional Information (per serving):

- Calories: 330
- Protein: 34g
- Carbohydrates: 6g
- Dietary Fiber: 3g
- Sugars: 2g
- Fat: 18g
- Saturated Fat: 3g
- Sodium: 70mg

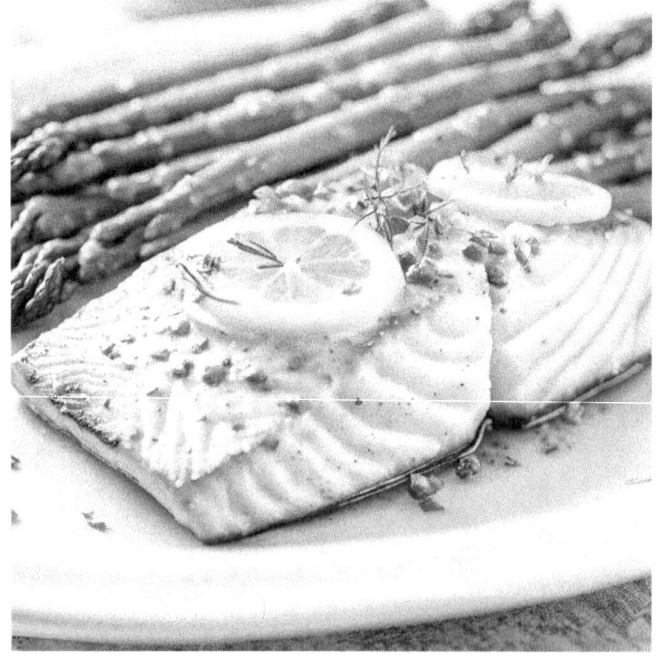

11. Seared Scallops with Spinach
Servings: 4
Cooking Time: 20 minutes
Ingredients:
- 1 pound sea scallops
- 2 tablespoons olive oil
- 3 cloves garlic, minced
- 1/4 cup low-sodium vegetable broth
- 1 tablespoon fresh lemon juice
- 6 cups fresh spinach

Instructions:
1. Pat the scallops dry with paper towels.
2. Heat 1 tablespoon of olive oil in a large skillet over medium-high heat.
3. Add the scallops and sear for about 2-3 minutes on each side until golden brown and cooked through. Remove scallops from the skillet and set aside.
4. In the same skillet, add the remaining tablespoon of olive oil and garlic. Sauté for about 1 minute until fragrant.
5. Add the vegetable broth and lemon juice, and bring to a simmer.
6. Add the spinach and cook until wilted, about 2-3 minutes.
7. Serve the seared scallops over the sautéed spinach.

Nutritional Information (per serving):
- Calories: 250
- Protein: 24g
- Carbohydrates: 6g
- Dietary Fiber: 3g
- Sugars: 1g
- Fat: 14g
- Saturated Fat: 2g
- Sodium: 270mg

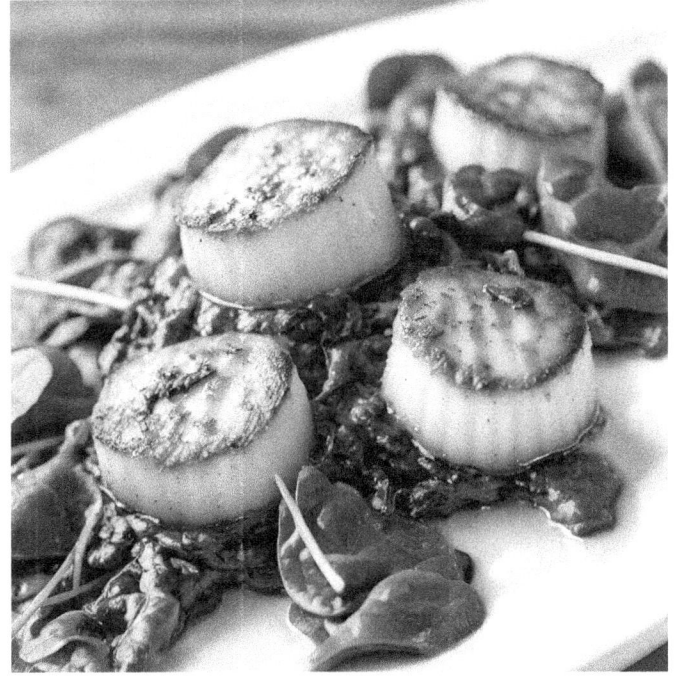

12. Cod with Tomato Basil Sauce

Servings: 4

Cooking Time: 25 minutes

Ingredients:

- 4 cod fillets (about 6 ounces each)
- 2 tablespoons olive oil
- 1 small onion, finely chopped
- 3 cloves garlic, minced
- 1 can (14.5 ounces) diced tomatoes
- 1/4 cup fresh basil, chopped
- 1 tablespoon fresh lemon juice

Instructions:

1. Preheat the oven to 375°F (190°C).
2. Heat the olive oil in a large skillet over medium heat.
3. Add the onion and garlic, and sauté for about 5 minutes until softened.
4. Add the diced tomatoes and bring to a simmer. Cook for about 5 minutes.
5. Stir in the chopped basil and lemon juice.
6. Place the cod fillets in a baking dish and pour the tomato basil sauce over them.
7. Bake for 15-20 minutes, or until the cod is cooked through and flakes easily with a fork.
8. Serve immediately.

Nutritional Information (per serving):

- Calories: 230
- Protein: 30g
- Carbohydrates: 8g
- Dietary Fiber: 2g
- Sugars: 5g
- Fat: 10g
- Saturated Fat: 1.5g
- Sodium: 300mg

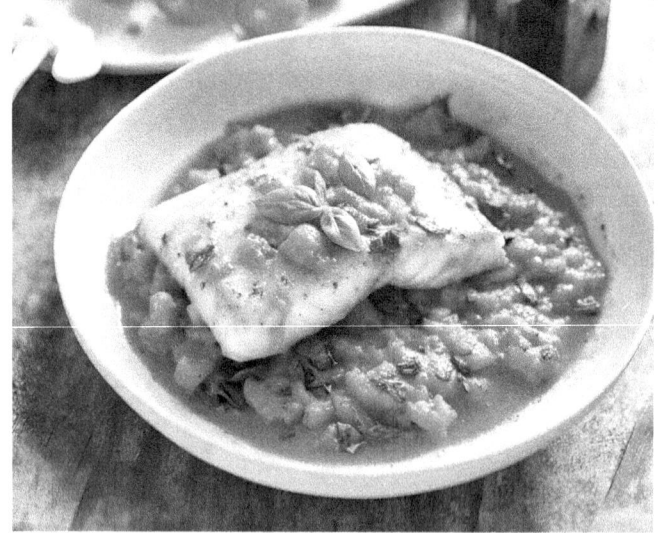

13. Salmon and Sweet Potato Cakes

Servings: 4 (8 cakes)
Cooking Time: 30 minutes
Ingredients:

- 1 pound cooked salmon, flaked
- 1 large sweet potato, cooked and mashed
- 1/4 cup plain Greek yogurt
- 1/4 cup chopped green onions
- 1 tablespoon Dijon mustard
- 1 egg, beaten
- 1/4 cup whole wheat breadcrumbs
- 2 tablespoons olive oil

Instructions:

1. In a large bowl, combine the flaked salmon, mashed sweet potato, Greek yogurt, green onions, Dijon mustard, and beaten egg. Mix well.
2. Stir in the breadcrumbs until well combined.
3. Form the mixture into 8 patties.
4. Heat the olive oil in a large skillet over medium heat.
5. Cook the patties for about 4-5 minutes on each side until golden brown and cooked through.
6. Serve immediately.

Nutritional Information (per serving):

- Calories: 320
- Protein: 25g
- Carbohydrates: 20g
- Dietary Fiber: 4g
- Sugars: 5g
- Fat: 16g
- Saturated Fat: 3g
- Sodium: 250mg

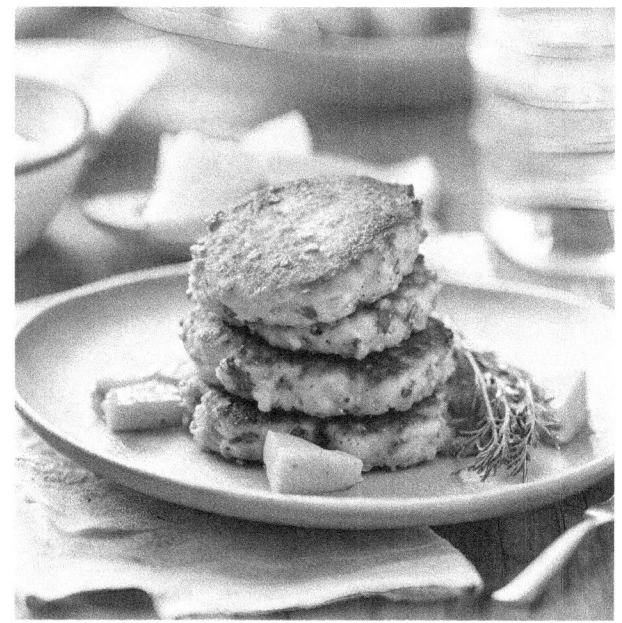

13. Lemon Herb Grilled Tuna

Servings: 4

Cooking Time: 20 minutes

Ingredients:

- 4 tuna steaks (about 6 ounces each)
- 3 tablespoons olive oil
- 2 tablespoons fresh lemon juice
- 2 teaspoons dried oregano
- 2 cloves garlic, minced
- 1 lemon, sliced into rounds

Instructions:

1. In a small bowl, mix the olive oil, lemon juice, oregano, and minced garlic.
2. Brush the tuna steaks with the olive oil mixture on both sides.
3. Preheat the grill to medium-high heat.
4. Grill the tuna steaks for about 4-5 minutes on each side or until cooked to your desired level of doneness.
5. Serve the tuna steaks with lemon slices on top.

Nutritional Information (per serving):

- Calories: 320
- Protein: 40g
- Carbohydrates: 1g
- Dietary Fiber: 0g
- Sugars: 0g
- Fat: 18g
- Saturated Fat: 3g
- Sodium: 60mg

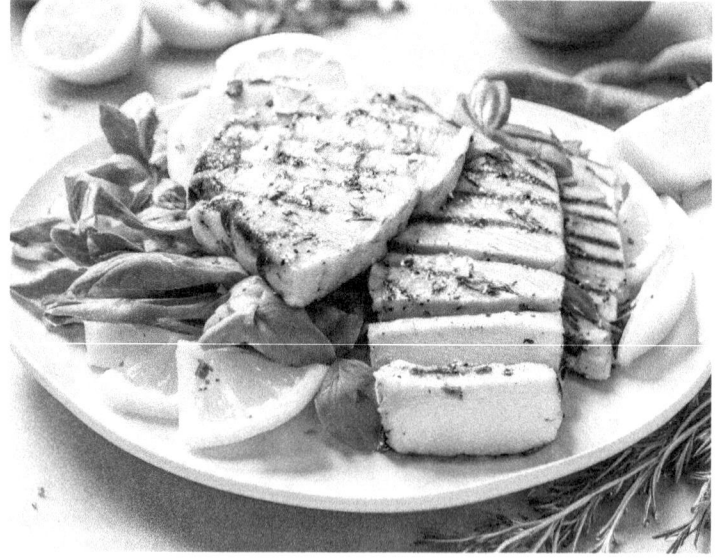

14. Tilapia with Mango Salsa
Servings: 4
Cooking Time: 20 minutes
Ingredients:

- 4 tilapia fillets (about 6 ounces each)
- 2 tablespoons olive oil
- 1 tablespoon lime juice
- 1 teaspoon cumin
- 1 mango, diced
- 1/4 cup red onion, finely chopped
- 1/4 cup red bell pepper, finely chopped
- 1 tablespoon fresh cilantro, chopped

Instructions:

1. Preheat the oven to 375°F (190°C).
2. In a small bowl, mix the olive oil, lime juice, and cumin.
3. Brush the tilapia fillets with the olive oil mixture on both sides.
4. Place the fillets in a baking dish and bake for 15 minutes or until the fish is cooked through and flakes easily with a fork.
5. In another bowl, combine the diced mango, red onion, red bell pepper, and cilantro to make the mango salsa.
6. Serve the tilapia topped with mango salsa.

Nutritional Information (per serving):

- Calories: 250
- Protein: 30g
- Carbohydrates: 12g
- Dietary Fiber: 2g
- Sugars: 9g
- Fat: 10g
- Saturated Fat: 1.5g
- Sodium: 60mg

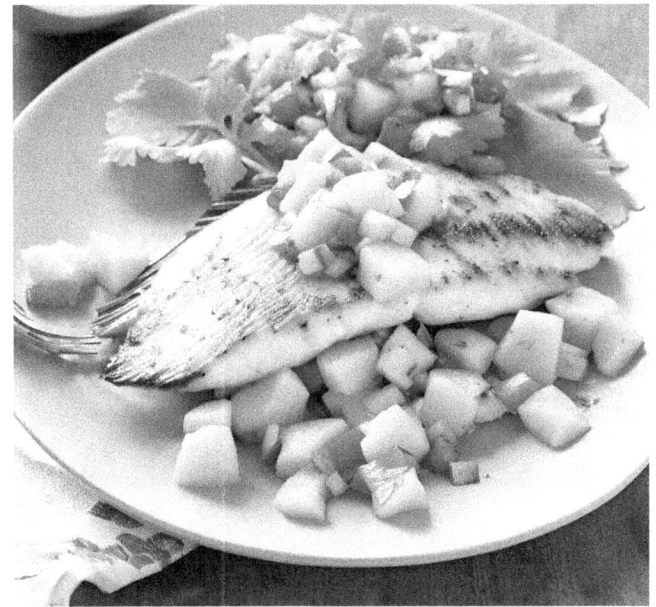

15. Fish and Vegetable Soup
Servings: 4
Cooking Time: 30 minutes
Ingredients:

- 1 pound white fish fillets (such as cod or halibut), cut into bite-sized pieces
- 1 tablespoon olive oil
- 1 onion, finely chopped
- 2 cloves garlic, minced
- 2 carrots, sliced
- 2 celery stalks, sliced
- 1 zucchini, diced
- 4 cups low-sodium vegetable broth
- 1 can (14.5 ounces) diced tomatoes
- 1 teaspoon dried thyme
- 1 teaspoon dried basil
- 1 tablespoon fresh lemon juice

Instructions:

1. Heat the olive oil in a large pot over medium heat.
2. Add the onion and garlic, and sauté for about 5 minutes until softened.
3. Add the carrots, celery, and zucchini, and cook for another 5 minutes.
4. Pour in the vegetable broth and diced tomatoes, and bring to a boil.
5. Add the dried thyme and basil, and simmer for 10 minutes.
6. Add the fish pieces and simmer for another 5 minutes, or until the fish is cooked through.
7. Stir in the lemon juice and serve hot.

Nutritional Information (per serving):

- Calories: 200
- Protein: 28g
- Carbohydrates: 12g
- Dietary Fiber: 3g
- Sugars: 6g
- Fat: 6g
- Saturated Fat: 1g
- Sodium: 250mg

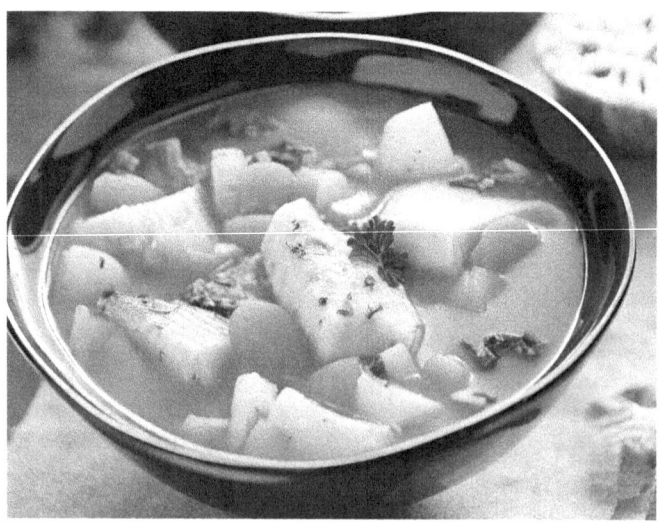

16. Grilled Salmon with Avocado Salsa
Servings: 4
Cooking Time: 20 minutes
Ingredients:

- 4 salmon fillets (about 6 ounces each)
- 2 tablespoons olive oil
- 2 tablespoons fresh lime juice
- 1 teaspoon ground cumin
- 1 avocado, diced
- 1/4 cup red onion, finely chopped
- 1/4 cup cherry tomatoes, halved
- 1 tablespoon fresh cilantro, chopped

Instructions:

1. In a small bowl, mix the olive oil, lime juice, and ground cumin.
2. Brush the salmon fillets with the olive oil mixture on both sides.
3. Preheat the grill to medium-high heat.
4. Grill the salmon fillets for about 5-7 minutes on each side, or until the salmon is cooked through and flakes easily with a fork.
5. In another bowl, combine the diced avocado, red onion, cherry tomatoes, and cilantro to make the avocado salsa.
6. Serve the grilled salmon topped with avocado salsa.

Nutritional Information (per serving):

- Calories: 370
- Protein: 35g
- Carbohydrates: 10g
- Dietary Fiber: 5g
- Sugars: 1g
- Fat: 22g
- Saturated Fat: 3g
- Sodium: 80mg

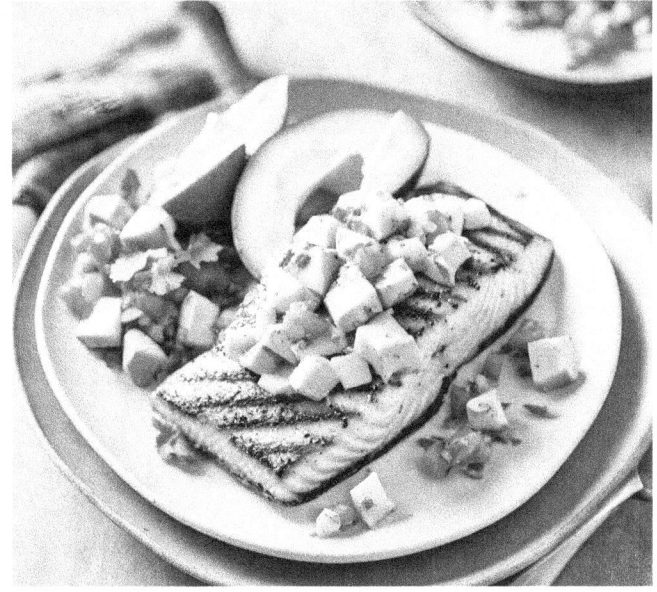

17. Baked Trout with Lemon and Thyme
Servings: 4
Cooking Time: 25 minutes
Ingredients:
- 4 trout fillets (about 6 ounces each)
- 2 tablespoons olive oil
- 2 tablespoons fresh lemon juice
- 1 teaspoon dried thyme
- 1 lemon, sliced into rounds

Instructions:
1. Preheat the oven to 375°F (190°C).
2. In a small bowl, mix the olive oil, lemon juice, and dried thyme.
3. Place the trout fillets in a baking dish.
4. Brush the olive oil mixture over the trout fillets.
5. Arrange the lemon slices on top of the fillets.
6. Bake for 15-20 minutes, or until the trout is cooked through and flakes easily with a fork.
7. Serve immediately.

Nutritional Information (per serving):
- Calories: 280
- Protein: 30g
- Carbohydrates: 1g
- Dietary Fiber: 0g
- Sugars: 0g
- Fat: 16g
- Saturated Fat: 3g
- Sodium: 60mg

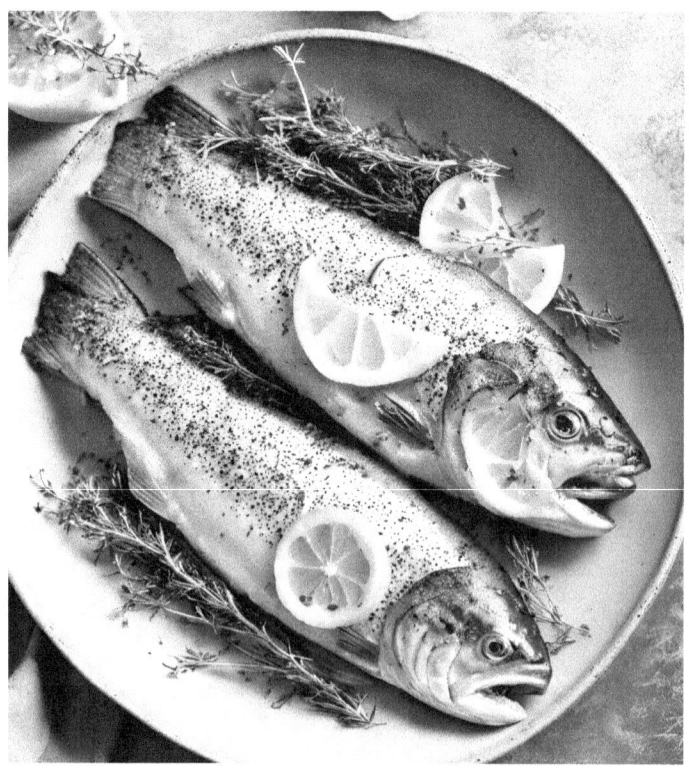

18. Tuna and White Bean Salad

Servings: 4
Cooking Time: 10 minutes
Ingredients:

- 2 cans tuna in water, drained
- 1 can (15 ounces) white beans, drained and rinsed
- 1/2 cup cherry tomatoes, halved
- 1/4 cup red onion, finely chopped
- 2 tablespoons fresh parsley, chopped
- 2 tablespoons olive oil
- 2 tablespoons fresh lemon juice

Instructions:

1. In a large bowl, combine the drained tuna, white beans, cherry tomatoes, red onion, and parsley.
2. In a small bowl, whisk together the olive oil and lemon juice.
3. Pour the dressing over the salad and toss gently to combine.
4. Serve immediately.

Nutritional Information (per serving):

- Calories: 300
- Protein: 28g
- Carbohydrates: 20g
- Dietary Fiber: 6g
- Sugars: 2g
- Fat: 12g
- Saturated Fat: 1.5g
- Sodium: 350mg

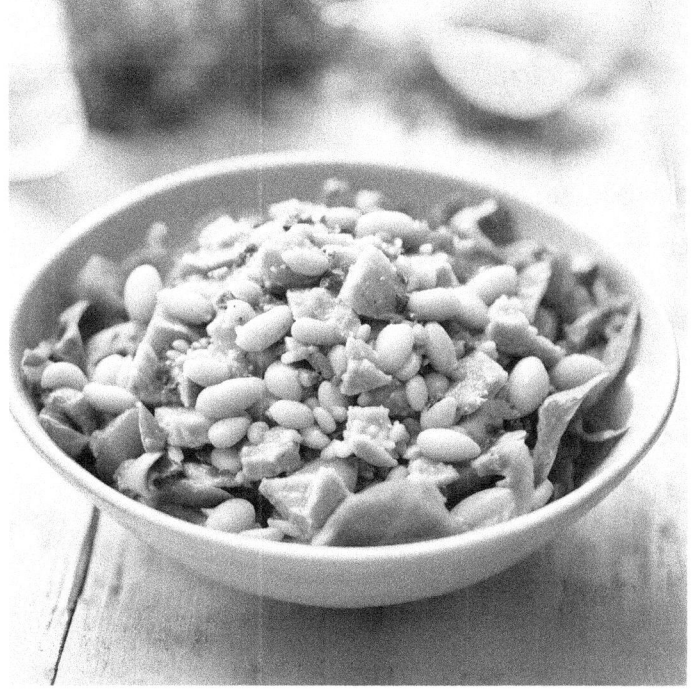

19. Salmon and Brown Rice Bowl
Servings: 4
Cooking Time: 30 minutes
Ingredients:

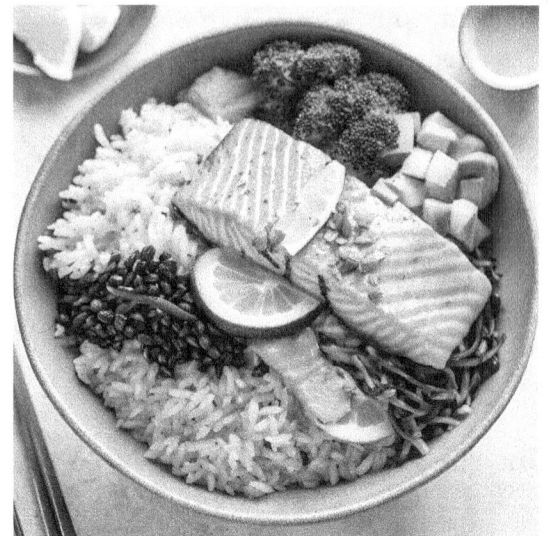

- 1 cup brown rice
- 2 cups water
- 4 salmon fillets (about 6 ounces each)
- 2 tablespoons olive oil
- 2 tablespoons fresh lemon juice
- 1 teaspoon dried oregano
- 1 avocado, sliced
- 1 cup steamed broccoli florets
- 1/2 cup shredded carrots
- 1/4 cup fresh parsley, chopped

Instructions:

1. In a medium saucepan, bring the water to a boil. Add the brown rice, reduce heat to low, cover, and simmer for 20 minutes or until the rice is cooked and the water is absorbed.
2. Preheat the oven to 375°F (190°C).
3. In a small bowl, mix the olive oil, lemon juice, and dried oregano.
4. Place the salmon fillets on a baking sheet lined with parchment paper. Brush the olive oil mixture over the salmon.
5. Bake the salmon for 15-20 minutes, or until the salmon is cooked through and flakes easily with a fork.
6. Divide the cooked brown rice among four bowls.
7. Top each bowl with a salmon fillet, avocado slices, steamed broccoli, shredded carrots, and chopped parsley.
8. Serve immediately.

Nutritional Information (per serving):

- Calories: 450
- Protein: 35g
- Carbohydrates: 30g
- Dietary Fiber: 8g
- Sugars: 3g
- Fat: 20g
- Saturated Fat: 3g
- Sodium: 120mg

20. Mediterranean Baked Cod

Servings: 4

Cooking Time: 30 minutes

Ingredients:

- 4 cod fillets (about 6 ounces each)
- 2 tablespoons olive oil
- 1 cup cherry tomatoes, halved
- 1/2 cup Kalamata olives, pitted and halved
- 1/4 cup red onion, thinly sliced
- 2 cloves garlic, minced
- 1 teaspoon dried oregano
- 1 tablespoon fresh lemon juice
- 1/4 cup fresh parsley, chopped

Instructions:

1. Preheat the oven to 375°F (190°C).
2. Place the cod fillets in a baking dish.
3. In a bowl, mix the olive oil, cherry tomatoes, olives, red onion, garlic, oregano, and lemon juice.
4. Pour the mixture over the cod fillets.
5. Bake for 20-25 minutes or until the cod is cooked through and flakes easily with a fork.
6. Garnish with chopped parsley and serve immediately.

Nutritional Information (per serving):

- Calories: 280
- Protein: 32g
- Carbohydrates: 6g
- Dietary Fiber: 2g
- Sugars: 2g
- Fat: 14g
- Saturated Fat: 2g
- Sodium: 200mg

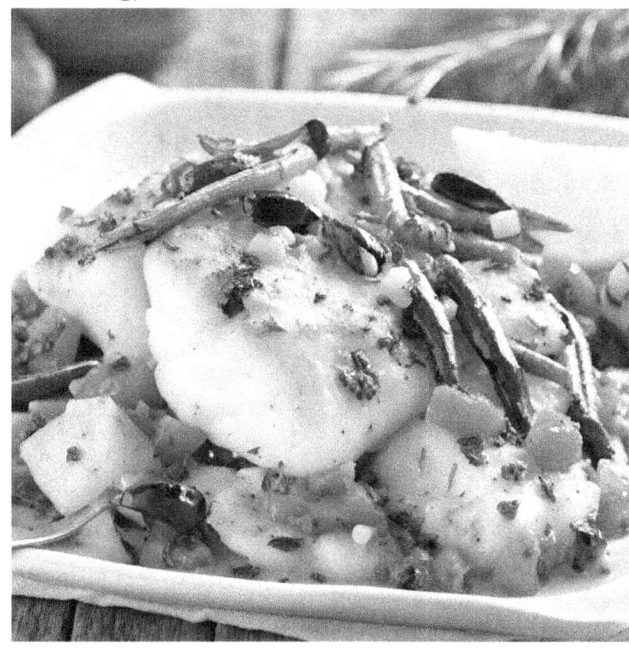

21. Ginger Soy Grilled Shrimp

Servings: 4

Cooking Time: 20 minutes

Ingredients:

- 1 pound shrimp, peeled and deveined
- 2 tablespoons soy sauce (low sodium)
- 1 tablespoon fresh ginger, grated
- 2 cloves garlic, minced
- 2 tablespoons olive oil
- 1 tablespoon honey
- 1 tablespoon fresh lime juice

Instructions:

1. In a bowl, mix the soy sauce, ginger, garlic, olive oil, honey, and lime juice.
2. Add the shrimp and marinate for at least 15 minutes.
3. Preheat the grill to medium-high heat.
4. Thread the shrimp onto skewers.
5. Grill the shrimp for about 2-3 minutes on each side until pink and cooked through.
6. Serve immediately.

Nutritional Information (per serving):

- Calories: 200
- Protein: 24g
- Carbohydrates: 6g
- Dietary Fiber: 0g
- Sugars: 4g
- Fat: 8g
- Saturated Fat: 1g
- Sodium: 500mg

22. Lemon Dill Tuna Steaks

Servings: 4
Cooking Time: 20 minutes
Ingredients:

- 4 tuna steaks (about 6 ounces each)
- 2 tablespoons olive oil
- 2 tablespoons fresh lemon juice
- 2 teaspoons dried dill
- 2 cloves garlic, minced

Instructions:

1. In a small bowl, mix the olive oil, lemon juice, dill, and garlic.
2. Brush the mixture over the tuna steaks.
3. Preheat the grill to medium-high heat.
4. Grill the tuna steaks for about 4-5 minutes on each side or until cooked to your desired level of doneness.
5. Serve immediately.

Nutritional Information (per serving):

- Calories: 310
- Protein: 40g
- Carbohydrates: 1g
- Dietary Fiber: 0g
- Sugars: 0g
- Fat: 16g
- Saturated Fat: 3g
- Sodium: 60mg

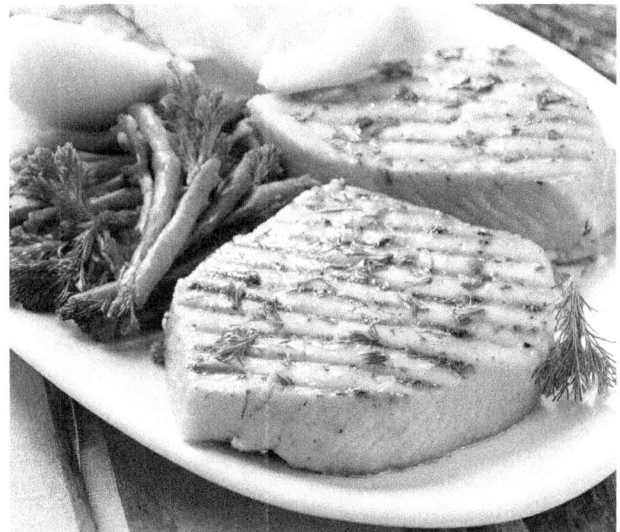

23. Broiled Tilapia with Fresh Salsa

Servings: 4

Cooking Time: 20 minutes

Ingredients:

- 4 tilapia fillets (about 6 ounces each)
- 2 tablespoons olive oil
- 1 tablespoon fresh lime juice
- 1 teaspoon cumin
- 1 cup diced tomatoes
- 1/4 cup red onion, finely chopped
- 1/4 cup cilantro, chopped
- 1 jalapeño, seeded and finely chopped

Instructions:

1. Preheat the broiler.
2. In a small bowl, mix the olive oil, lime juice, and cumin.
3. Brush the mixture over the tilapia fillets.
4. Broil the tilapia for about 4-5 minutes on each side or until cooked through.
5. In another bowl, mix the tomatoes, red onion, cilantro, and jalapeño to make the salsa.
6. Serve the tilapia topped with the fresh salsa.

Nutritional Information (per serving):

- Calories: 240
- Protein: 30g
- Carbohydrates: 6g
- Dietary Fiber: 2g
- Sugars: 3g
- Fat: 10g
- Saturated Fat: 1.5g
- Sodium: 90mg

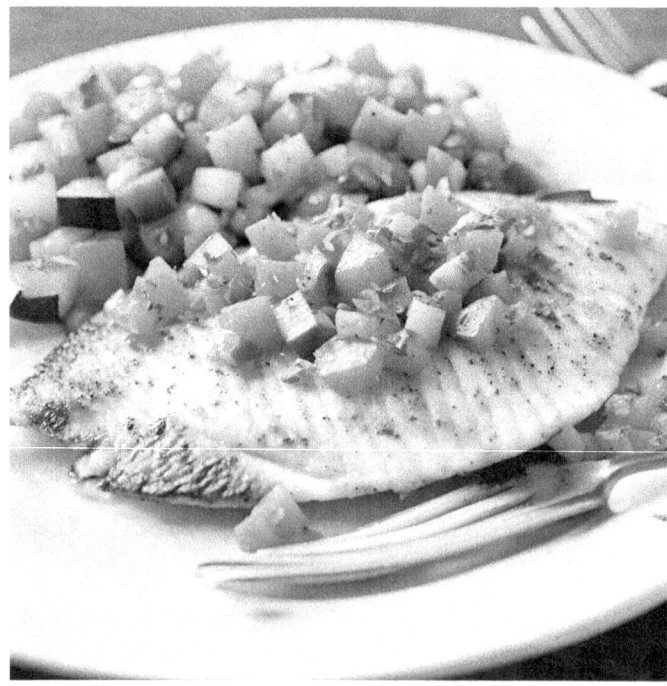

24. Garlic Butter Salmon
Servings: 4
Cooking Time: 20 minutes
Ingredients:
- 4 salmon fillets (about 6 ounces each)
- 3 tablespoons olive oil
- 2 tablespoons fresh lemon juice
- 4 cloves garlic, minced
- 1 tablespoon fresh parsley, chopped

Instructions:
1. Preheat the oven to 375°F (190°C).
2. In a small bowl, mix the olive oil, lemon juice, and minced garlic.
3. Place the salmon fillets in a baking dish.
4. Pour the garlic mixture over the salmon fillets.
5. Bake for 15-20 minutes or until the salmon is cooked through and flakes easily with a fork.
6. Garnish with chopped parsley and serve immediately.

Nutritional Information (per serving):
- Calories: 350
- Protein: 35g
- Carbohydrates: 2g
- Dietary Fiber: 0g
- Sugars: 0g
- Fat: 22g
- Saturated Fat: 3g
- Sodium: 70mg

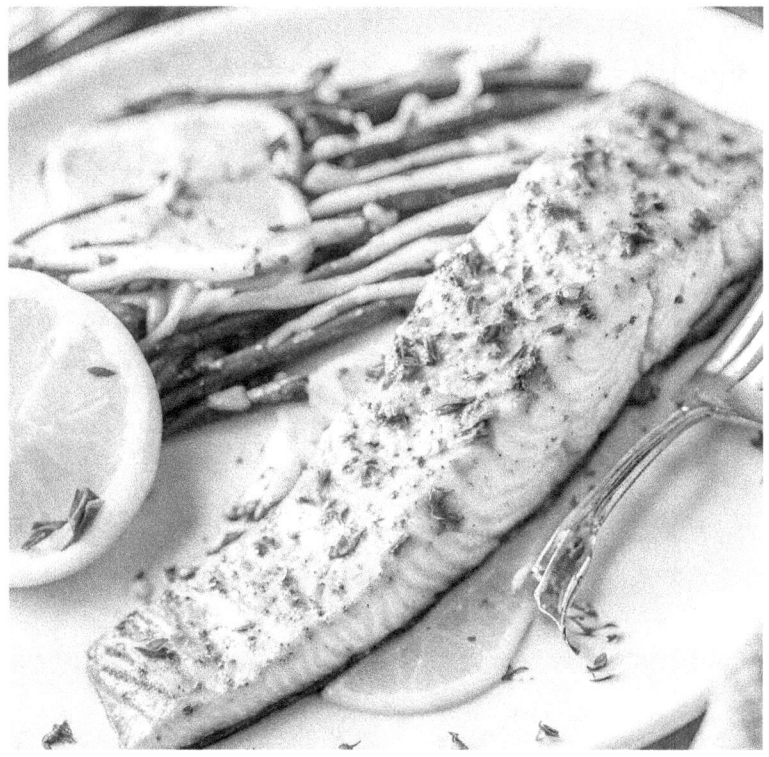

25. Baked Sole with Lemon and Capers
Servings: 4
Cooking Time: 20 minutes
Ingredients:
- 4 sole fillets (about 6 ounces each)
- 2 tablespoons olive oil
- 2 tablespoons fresh lemon juice
- 1 tablespoon capers, drained and rinsed
- 1 lemon, sliced into rounds

Instructions:
1. Preheat the oven to 375°F (190°C).
2. In a small bowl, mix the olive oil, lemon juice, and capers.
3. Place the sole fillets in a baking dish.
4. Pour the olive oil mixture over the sole fillets.
5. Arrange the lemon slices on top of the fillets.
6. Bake for 15-20 minutes or until the sole is cooked through and flakes easily with a fork.
7. Serve immediately.

Nutritional Information (per serving):
- Calories: 220
- Protein: 30g
- Carbohydrates: 2g
- Dietary Fiber: 0g
- Sugars: 0g
- Fat: 10g
- Saturated Fat: 1.5g
- Sodium: 180mg

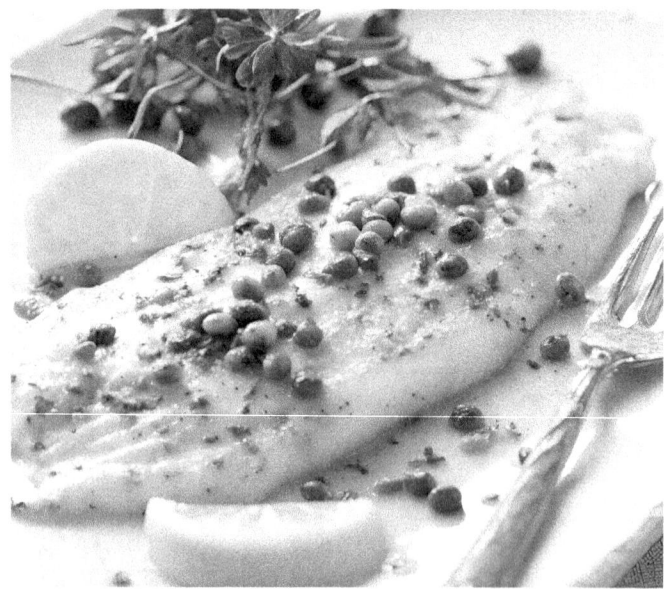

26. Seared Ahi Tuna Salad

Servings: 4
Cooking Time: 15 minutes
Ingredients:

- 4 ahi tuna steaks (about 6 ounces each)
- 2 tablespoons olive oil
- 1 tablespoon sesame oil
- 2 tablespoons soy sauce (low sodium)
- 1 tablespoon fresh lime juice
- 6 cups mixed greens
- 1 avocado, sliced
- 1 cup cherry tomatoes, halved
- 1/4 cup red onion, thinly sliced

Instructions:

1. In a small bowl, mix the olive oil, sesame oil, soy sauce, and lime juice.
2. Brush the mixture over the ahi tuna steaks.
3. Heat a non-stick skillet over medium-high heat.
4. Sear the tuna steaks for about 2 minutes on each side or until desired doneness.
5. In a large bowl, combine the mixed greens, avocado, cherry tomatoes, and red onion.
6. Top with the seared ahi tuna and serve immediately.

Nutritional Information (per serving):

- Calories: 350
- Protein: 38g
- Carbohydrates: 10g
- Dietary Fiber: 5g
- Sugars: 2g
- Fat: 18g
- Saturated Fat: 3g
- Sodium: 300mg

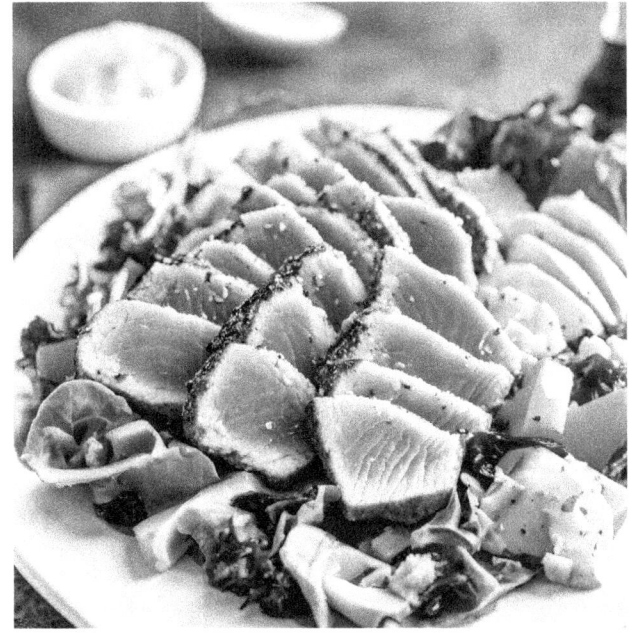

27. Baked Salmon with Pesto

Servings: 4

Cooking Time: 20 minutes

Ingredients:

- 4 salmon fillets (about 6 ounces each)
- 4 tablespoons prepared pesto
- 2 tablespoons olive oil
- 1 tablespoon fresh lemon juice

Instructions:

1. Preheat the oven to 375°F (190°C).
2. In a small bowl, mix the olive oil and lemon juice.
3. Place the salmon fillets in a baking dish.
4. Brush the olive oil mixture over the salmon fillets.
5. Spread 1 tablespoon of pesto over each salmon fillet.
6. Bake for 15-20 minutes or until the salmon is cooked through and flakes easily with a fork.
7. Serve immediately.

Nutritional Information (per serving):

- Calories: 380
- Protein: 35g
- Carbohydrates: 2g
- Dietary Fiber: 0g
- Sugars: 0g
- Fat: 24g
- Saturated Fat: 4g
- Sodium: 220mg

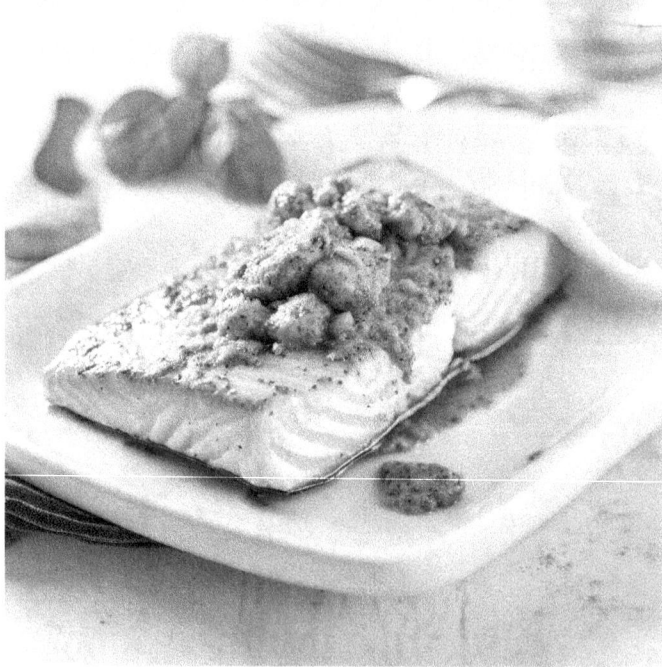

28. Sesame Crusted Tuna

Servings: 4
Cooking Time: 20 minutes
Ingredients:

- 4 tuna steaks (about 6 ounces each)
- 2 tablespoons soy sauce (low sodium)
- 1 tablespoon sesame oil
- 1 tablespoon fresh ginger, grated
- 2 tablespoons sesame seeds
- 1 tablespoon olive oil

Instructions:

1. In a small bowl, mix the soy sauce, sesame oil, and grated ginger.
2. Marinate the tuna steaks in the mixture for at least 15 minutes.
3. Press the sesame seeds onto both sides of the tuna steaks.
4. Heat the olive oil in a non-stick skillet over medium-high heat.
5. Sear the tuna steaks for about 2 minutes on each side or until desired doneness.
6. Serve immediately.

Nutritional Information (per serving):

- Calories: 320
- Protein: 40g
- Carbohydrates: 2g
- Dietary Fiber: 1g
- Sugars: 0g
- Fat: 18g
- Saturated Fat: 3g
- Sodium: 300mg

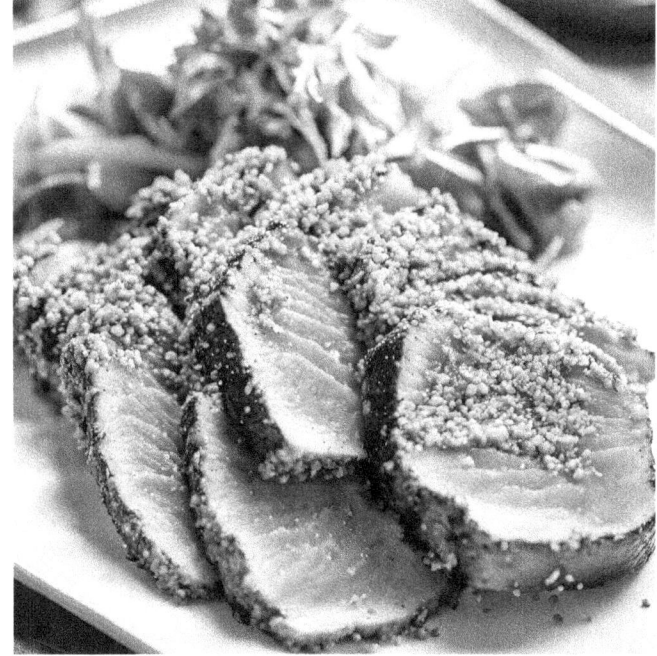

Poultry Recipes

1. Grilled Lemon Herb Chicken
Servings: 4
Cooking Time: 20 minutes (plus marinating time)
Ingredients:

- 4 boneless, skinless chicken breasts
- 1/4 cup olive oil
- 2 tablespoons fresh lemon juice
- 2 cloves garlic, minced
- 1 tablespoon fresh rosemary, chopped
- 1 tablespoon fresh thyme, chopped
- 1 tablespoon fresh parsley, chopped
- 1 lemon, sliced into rounds

Instructions:

1. In a small bowl, mix the olive oil, lemon juice, garlic, rosemary, thyme, and parsley.
2. Place the chicken breasts in a resealable plastic bag and pour the marinade over them. Seal the bag and refrigerate for at least 30 minutes, preferably 2-4 hours.
3. Preheat the grill to medium-high heat.
4. Remove the chicken from the marinade and discard the marinade.
5. Grill the chicken breasts for about 6-7 minutes on each side, or until the internal temperature reaches 165°F (74°C).
6. Serve the chicken with lemon slices on top.

Nutritional Information (per serving):

- Calories: 300
- Protein: 32g
- Carbohydrates: 2g
- Dietary Fiber: 0g
- Sugars: 0g
- Fat: 18g
- Saturated Fat: 2.5g
- Sodium: 70mg

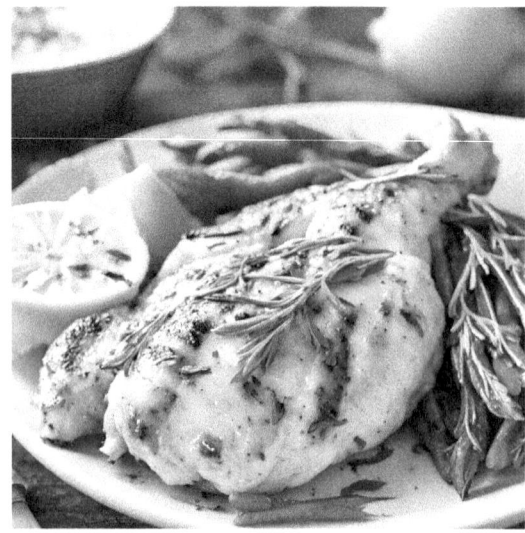

2. Baked Chicken with Rosemary and Garlic

Servings: 4

Cooking Time: 40 minutes

Ingredients:

- 4 boneless, skinless chicken breasts
- 2 tablespoons olive oil
- 4 cloves garlic, minced
- 1 tablespoon fresh rosemary, chopped
- 1 tablespoon fresh lemon juice
- 1 lemon, sliced into rounds

Instructions:

1. Preheat the oven to 375°F (190°C).
2. In a small bowl, mix the olive oil, garlic, rosemary, and lemon juice.
3. Place the chicken breasts in a baking dish and brush the olive oil mixture over them.
4. Arrange the lemon slices on top of the chicken.
5. Bake for 30-35 minutes, or until the chicken is cooked through and the internal temperature reaches 165°F (74°C).
6. Serve immediately.

Nutritional Information (per serving):

- Calories: 290
- Protein: 32g
- Carbohydrates: 2g
- Dietary Fiber: 0g
- Sugars: 0g
- Fat: 17g
- Saturated Fat: 2.5g
- Sodium: 70mg

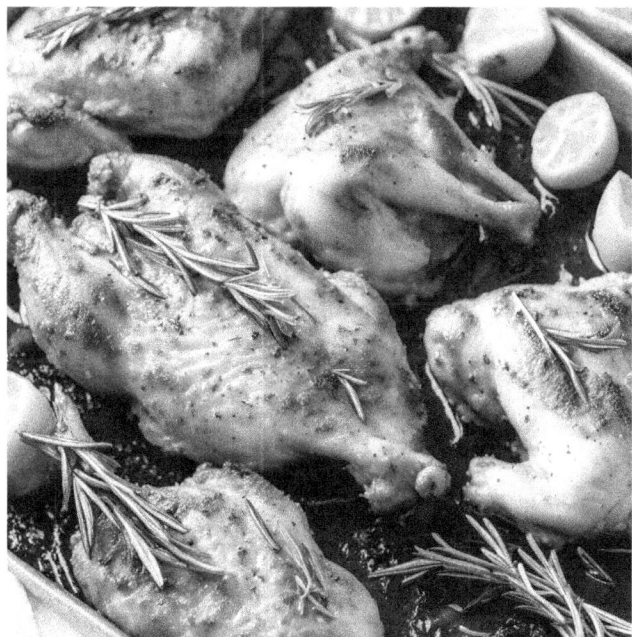

3. Chicken and Vegetable Stir-Fry

Servings: 4
Cooking Time: 20 minutes
Ingredients:

- 1 pound boneless, skinless chicken breasts, cut into strips
- 2 tablespoons olive oil
- 1 red bell pepper, sliced
- 1 yellow bell pepper, sliced
- 1 zucchini, sliced
- 1 carrot, julienned
- 2 cloves garlic, minced
- 1 tablespoon fresh ginger, grated
- 2 tablespoons soy sauce (low sodium)
- 1 tablespoon honey
- 1 tablespoon sesame oil
- 1/4 cup green onions, sliced

Instructions:

1. Heat the olive oil in a large skillet or wok over medium-high heat.
2. Add the chicken strips and cook for about 5-6 minutes, or until the chicken is browned and cooked through. Remove the chicken from the skillet and set aside.
3. In the same skillet, add the garlic and ginger and sauté for about 1 minute until fragrant.
4. Add the bell peppers, zucchini, and carrot to the skillet and stir-fry for about 5-6 minutes until the vegetables are tender-crisp.
5. In a small bowl, mix the soy sauce, honey, and sesame oil.
6. Return the chicken to the skillet and pour the soy sauce mixture over the chicken and vegetables. Stir to combine and cook for another 2-3 minutes until heated through.
7. Garnish with sliced green onions and serve immediately.

Nutritional Information (per serving):

- Calories: 280
- Protein: 28g
- Carbohydrates: 15g
- Dietary Fiber: 3g
- Sugars: 8g
- Fat: 12g
- Saturated Fat: 2g
- Sodium: 350mg

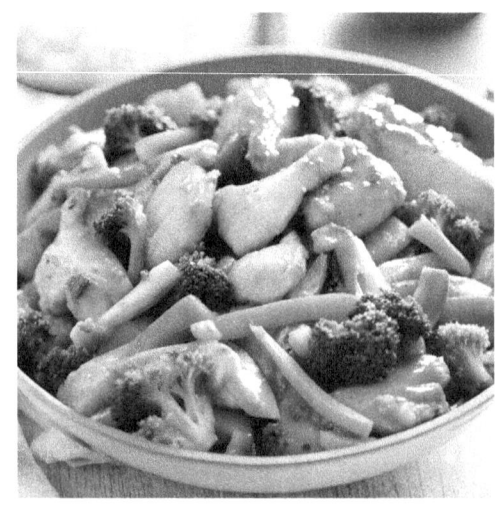

4. Lemon Pepper Chicken

Servings: 4
Cooking Time: 30 minutes
Ingredients:

- 4 boneless, skinless chicken breasts
- 3 tablespoons olive oil
- 2 tablespoons fresh lemon juice
- 1 tablespoon lemon zest
- 2 cloves garlic, minced
- 1 tablespoon freshly ground black pepper

Instructions:

1. Preheat the oven to 375°F (190°C).
2. In a small bowl, mix the olive oil, lemon juice, lemon zest, garlic, and black pepper.
3. Place the chicken breasts in a baking dish and brush the olive oil mixture over them.
4. Bake for 25-30 minutes, or until the chicken is cooked through and the internal temperature reaches 165°F (74°C).
5. Serve immediately.

Nutritional Information (per serving):

- Calories: 280
- Protein: 32g
- Carbohydrates: 1g
- Dietary Fiber: 0g
- Sugars: 0g
- Fat: 16g
- Saturated Fat: 2g
- Sodium: 70mg

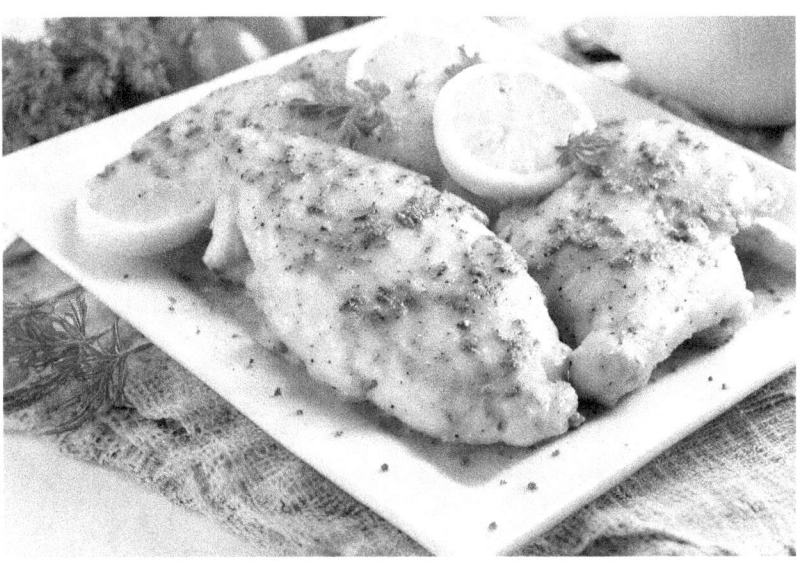

5. Herb Roasted Chicken
Servings: 4
Cooking Time: 1 hour
Ingredients:
- 1 whole chicken (about 4 pounds)
- 1/4 cup olive oil
- 2 tablespoons fresh rosemary, chopped
- 2 tablespoons fresh thyme, chopped
- 2 tablespoons fresh parsley, chopped
- 3 cloves garlic, minced
- 1 lemon, halved

Instructions:
1. Preheat the oven to 375°F (190°C).
2. In a small bowl, mix the olive oil, rosemary, thyme, parsley, and garlic.
3. Rub the herb mixture all over the chicken, including under the skin.
4. Place the lemon halves inside the cavity of the chicken.
5. Place the chicken in a roasting pan and roast for about 1 hour, or until the internal temperature reaches 165°F (74°C).
6. Let the chicken rest for 10 minutes before carving and serving.

Nutritional Information (per serving):
- Calories: 450
- Protein: 36g
- Carbohydrates: 1g
- Dietary Fiber: 0g
- Sugars: 0g
- Fat: 32g
- Saturated Fat: 8g
- Sodium: 90mg

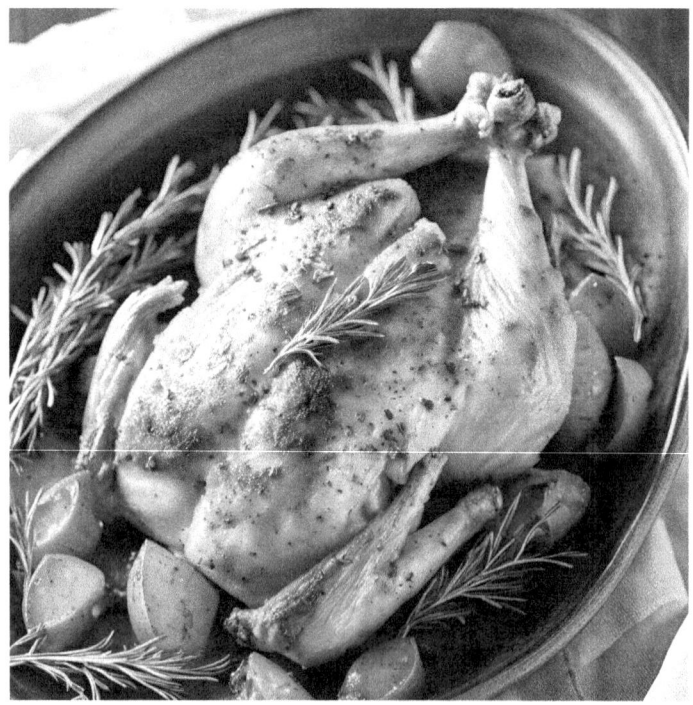

6. Stuffed Chicken Breast

Servings: 4
Cooking Time: 40 minutes
Ingredients:

- 4 boneless, skinless chicken breasts
- 1/2 cup fresh spinach, chopped
- 1/2 cup ricotta cheese
- 1/4 cup sun-dried tomatoes, chopped
- 2 tablespoons olive oil
- 2 cloves garlic, minced
- 1 teaspoon dried basil

Instructions:

1. Preheat the oven to 375°F (190°C).
2. In a small bowl, mix the spinach, ricotta cheese, sun-dried tomatoes, garlic, and dried basil.
3. Using a sharp knife, cut a pocket into the side of each chicken breast.
4. Stuff each pocket with the spinach mixture.
5. Secure the openings with toothpicks if necessary.
6. Heat the olive oil in a large oven-safe skillet over medium-high heat.
7. Sear the stuffed chicken breasts for about 3-4 minutes on each side until golden brown.
8. Transfer the skillet to the oven and bake for 20-25 minutes, or until the chicken is cooked through and the internal temperature reaches 165°F (74°C).
9. Serve immediately.

Nutritional Information (per serving):

- Calories: 350
- Protein: 38g
- Carbohydrates: 4g
- Dietary Fiber: 1g
- Sugars: 1g
- Fat: 18g
- Saturated Fat: 6g
- Sodium: 200mg

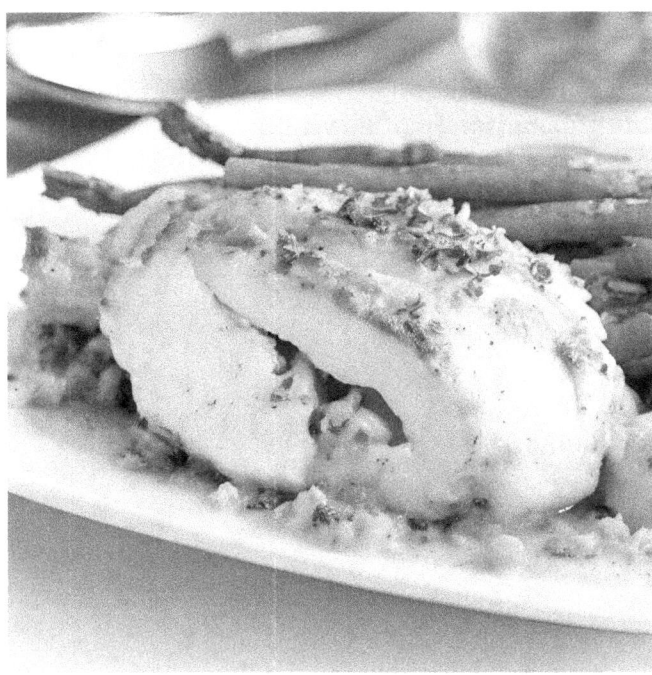

7. Chicken and Asparagus Stir-Fry
Servings: 4
Cooking Time: 20 minutes
Ingredients:

- 1 pound boneless, skinless chicken breasts, cut into thin strips
- 2 tablespoons olive oil
- 1 bunch asparagus, trimmed and cut into 2-inch pieces
- 1 red bell pepper, sliced
- 1 yellow bell pepper, sliced
- 3 cloves garlic, minced
- 1 tablespoon fresh ginger, grated
- 2 tablespoons soy sauce (low sodium)
- 1 tablespoon honey
- 1 tablespoon sesame oil
- 1/4 cup sliced green onions

Instructions:

1. Heat the olive oil in a large skillet or wok over medium-high heat.
2. Add the chicken strips and cook for about 5-6 minutes until browned and cooked through. Remove the chicken from the skillet and set aside.
3. In the same skillet, add the garlic and ginger, and sauté for about 1 minute until fragrant.
4. Add the asparagus and bell peppers to the skillet and stir-fry for about 5-6 minutes until the vegetables are tender-crisp.
5. In a small bowl, mix the soy sauce, honey, and sesame oil.
6. Return the chicken to the skillet and pour the soy sauce mixture over the chicken and vegetables. Stir to combine and cook for another 2-3 minutes until heated through.
7. Garnish with sliced green onions and serve immediately.

Nutritional Information (per serving):

- Calories: 280
- Protein: 26g
- Carbohydrates: 14g
- Dietary Fiber: 4g
- Sugars: 7g
- Fat: 14g
- Saturated Fat: 2g
- Sodium: 360mg

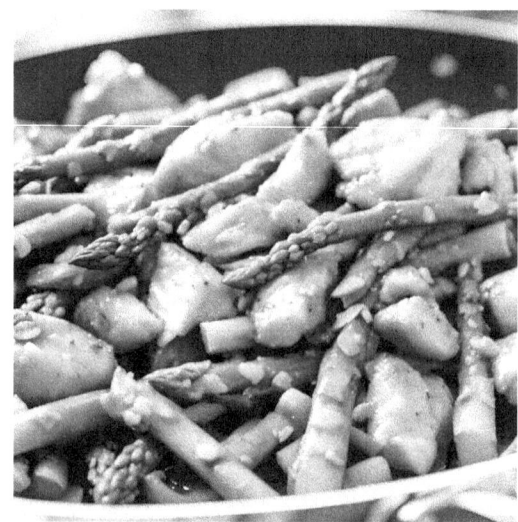

8. Chicken and Mango Salad

Servings: 4
Cooking Time: 20 minutes
Ingredients:

- 1 pound boneless, skinless chicken breasts, grilled and sliced
- 2 ripe mangoes, peeled and diced
- 1 red bell pepper, diced
- 1/2 red onion, thinly sliced
- 4 cups mixed greens (spinach, arugula, kale)
- 1/4 cup fresh cilantro, chopped
- 1/4 cup chopped cashews (optional)
- 2 tablespoons olive oil
- 2 tablespoons fresh lime juice
- 1 tablespoon honey
- 1 teaspoon Dijon mustard

Instructions:

1. In a large bowl, combine the grilled chicken, diced mangoes, red bell pepper, red onion, mixed greens, cilantro, and cashews (if using).
2. In a small bowl, whisk together the olive oil, lime juice, honey, and Dijon mustard to make the dressing.
3. Pour the dressing over the salad and toss gently to combine.
4. Serve immediately.

Nutritional Information (per serving):

- Calories: 350
- Protein: 28g
- Carbohydrates: 25g
- Dietary Fiber: 4g
- Sugars: 20g
- Fat: 16g
- Saturated Fat: 2g
- Sodium: 120mg

9. Chicken and Broccoli Bake

Servings: 4

Cooking Time: 40 minutes

Ingredients:

- 1 pound boneless, skinless chicken breasts, cubed
- 2 tablespoons olive oil
- 4 cups broccoli florets
- 1/2 cup low-sodium chicken broth
- 1/2 cup plain Greek yogurt
- 1/4 cup grated Parmesan cheese
- 1 teaspoon dried thyme
- 1/2 teaspoon garlic powder

Instructions:

1. Preheat the oven to 375°F (190°C).
2. Heat the olive oil in a large skillet over medium-high heat.
3. Add the chicken cubes and cook for about 5-6 minutes until browned and cooked through. Remove from heat and set aside.
4. In a large mixing bowl, combine the cooked chicken, broccoli florets, chicken broth, Greek yogurt, Parmesan cheese, thyme, and garlic powder. Mix well.
5. Transfer the mixture to a baking dish and spread evenly.
6. Bake for 25-30 minutes until the broccoli is tender and the top is golden brown.
7. Serve immediately.

Nutritional Information (per serving):

- Calories: 320
- Protein: 34g
- Carbohydrates: 12g
- Dietary Fiber: 4g
- Sugars: 4g
- Fat: 16g
- Saturated Fat: 4g
- Sodium: 200mg

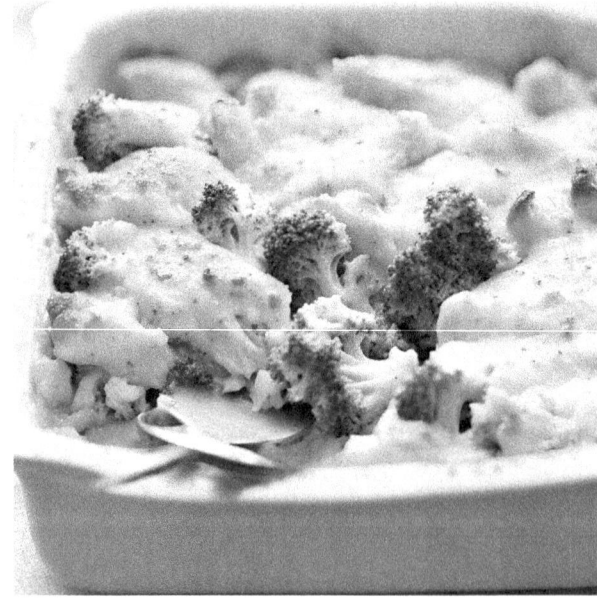

10. Garlic Lime Chicken

Servings: 4

Cooking Time: 30 minutes

Ingredients:

- 4 boneless, skinless chicken breasts
- 3 tablespoons olive oil
- 2 tablespoons fresh lime juice
- 3 cloves garlic, minced
- 1 teaspoon ground cumin
- 1 teaspoon paprika
- 1/4 cup fresh cilantro, chopped (optional)

Instructions:

1. Preheat the oven to 375°F (190°C).
2. In a small bowl, mix the olive oil, lime juice, garlic, cumin, and paprika.
3. Place the chicken breasts in a baking dish and brush the olive oil mixture over them.
4. Bake for 25-30 minutes, or until the chicken is cooked through and the internal temperature reaches 165°F (74°C).
5. Garnish with chopped cilantro (if using) and serve immediately.

Nutritional Information (per serving):

- Calories: 280
- Protein: 32g
- Carbohydrates: 2g
- Dietary Fiber: 0g
- Sugars: 0g
- Fat: 16g
- Saturated Fat: 2.5g
- Sodium: 70mg

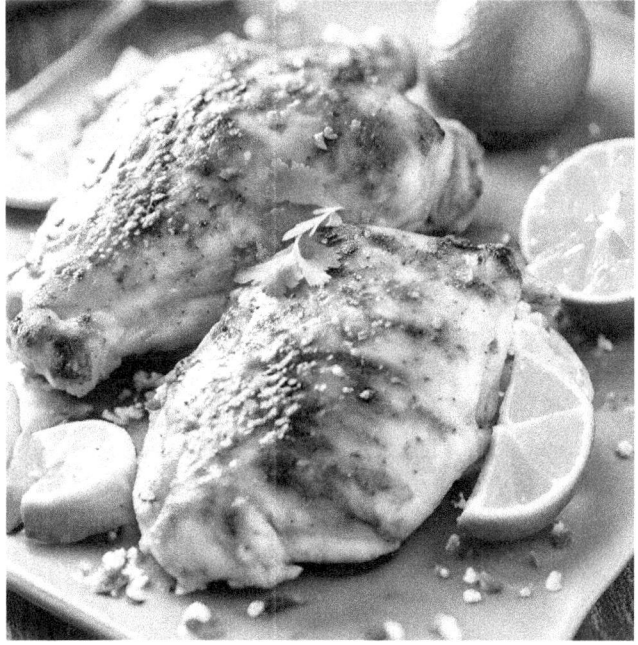

11. Chicken and Vegetable Kebabs

Servings: 4

Cooking Time: 30 minutes (plus marinating time)

Ingredients:

- 1 pound boneless, skinless chicken breasts, cut into 1-inch cubes
- 1 red bell pepper, cut into 1-inch pieces
- 1 yellow bell pepper, cut into 1-inch pieces
- 1 zucchini, sliced into 1/2-inch rounds
- 1 red onion, cut into wedges
- 2 tablespoons olive oil
- 2 tablespoons fresh lemon juice
- 2 cloves garlic, minced
- 1 teaspoon dried oregano

Instructions:

1. In a large bowl, mix the olive oil, lemon juice, garlic, and oregano.
2. Add the chicken cubes to the bowl and toss to coat. Marinate for at least 30 minutes in the refrigerator.
3. Preheat the grill to medium-high heat.
4. Thread the chicken and vegetables alternately onto skewers.
5. Grill the kebabs for about 10-12 minutes, turning occasionally, until the chicken is cooked through and the vegetables are tender.
6. Serve immediately.

Nutritional Information (per serving):

- Calories: 250
- Protein: 30g
- Carbohydrates: 10g
- Dietary Fiber: 3g
- Sugars: 4g
- Fat: 10g
- Saturated Fat: 1.5g
- Sodium: 70mg

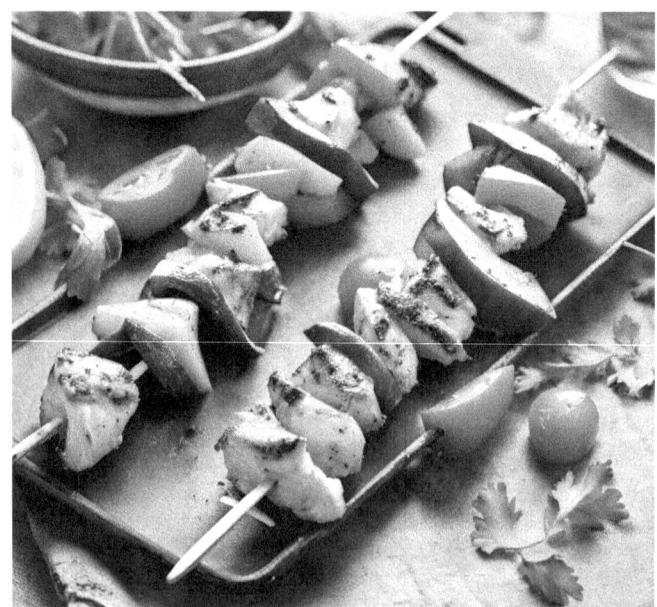

12. Honey Mustard Chicken

Servings: 4
Cooking Time: 30 minutes
Ingredients:

- 4 boneless, skinless chicken breasts
- 3 tablespoons Dijon mustard
- 2 tablespoons honey
- 2 tablespoons olive oil
- 2 cloves garlic, minced
- 1 tablespoon fresh lemon juice

Instructions:

1. Preheat the oven to 375°F (190°C).
2. In a small bowl, mix the Dijon mustard, honey, olive oil, garlic, and lemon juice.
3. Place the chicken breasts in a baking dish and brush the honey mustard mixture over them.
4. Bake for 25-30 minutes, or until the chicken is cooked through and the internal temperature reaches 165°F (74°C).
5. Serve immediately.

Nutritional Information (per serving):

- Calories: 290
- Protein: 32g
- Carbohydrates: 10g
- Dietary Fiber: 0g
- Sugars: 8g
- Fat: 12g
- Saturated Fat: 2g
- Sodium: 250mg

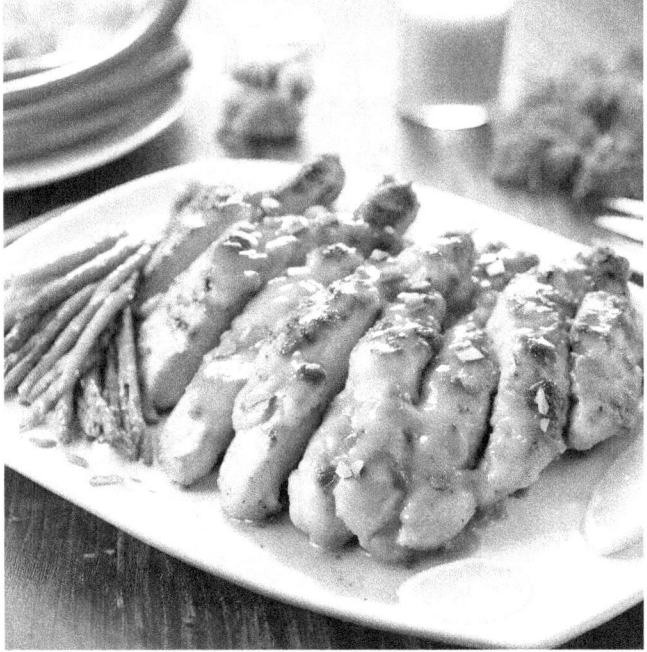

13. Chicken and Cauliflower Rice Stir-Fry
Servings: 4
Cooking Time: 20 minutes
Ingredients:
- 1 pound boneless, skinless chicken breasts, cut into thin strips
- 2 tablespoons olive oil
- 1 small head of cauliflower, grated into rice-sized pieces
- 1 red bell pepper, sliced
- 1 yellow bell pepper, sliced
- 1 cup snap peas
- 3 cloves garlic, minced
- 1 tablespoon fresh ginger, grated
- 2 tablespoons soy sauce (low sodium)
- 1 tablespoon sesame oil
- 1/4 cup green onions, sliced

Instructions:
1. Heat the olive oil in a large skillet or wok over medium-high heat.
2. Add the chicken strips and cook for about 5-6 minutes until browned and cooked through. Remove the chicken from the skillet and set aside.
3. In the same skillet, add the garlic and ginger and sauté for about 1 minute until fragrant.
4. Add the cauliflower rice, bell peppers, and snap peas to the skillet and stir-fry for about 5-6 minutes until the vegetables are tender-crisp.
5. In a small bowl, mix the soy sauce and sesame oil.
6. Return the chicken to the skillet and pour the soy sauce mixture over the chicken and vegetables. Stir to combine and cook for another 2-3 minutes until heated through.
7. Garnish with sliced green onions and serve immediately.

Nutritional Information (per serving):
- Calories: 250
- Protein: 28g
- Carbohydrates: 12g
- Dietary Fiber: 4g
- Sugars: 5g
- Fat: 10g
- Saturated Fat: 1.5g
- Sodium: 360mg

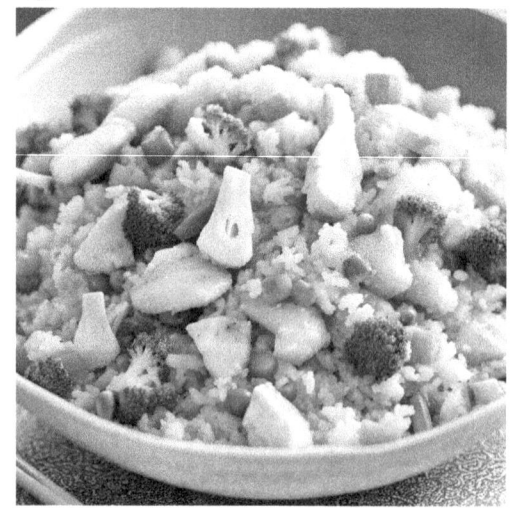

14. Cilantro Lime Chicken

Servings: 4

Cooking Time: 30 minutes (plus marinating time)

Ingredients:

- 4 boneless, skinless chicken breasts
- 1/4 cup olive oil
- 2 tablespoons fresh lime juice
- 2 cloves garlic, minced
- 1/4 cup fresh cilantro, chopped
- 1 teaspoon ground cumin

Instructions:

1. In a large bowl, mix the olive oil, lime juice, garlic, cilantro, and cumin.
2. Add the chicken breasts to the bowl and toss to coat. Marinate for at least 30 minutes in the refrigerator.
3. Preheat the grill to medium-high heat.
4. Remove the chicken from the marinade and discard the marinade.
5. Grill the chicken breasts for about 6-7 minutes on each side, or until the internal temperature reaches 165°F (74°C).
6. Serve immediately.

Nutritional Information (per serving):

- Calories: 280
- Protein: 32g
- Carbohydrates: 2g
- Dietary Fiber: 0g
- Sugars: 0g
- Fat: 16g
- Saturated Fat: 2.5g
- Sodium: 70mg

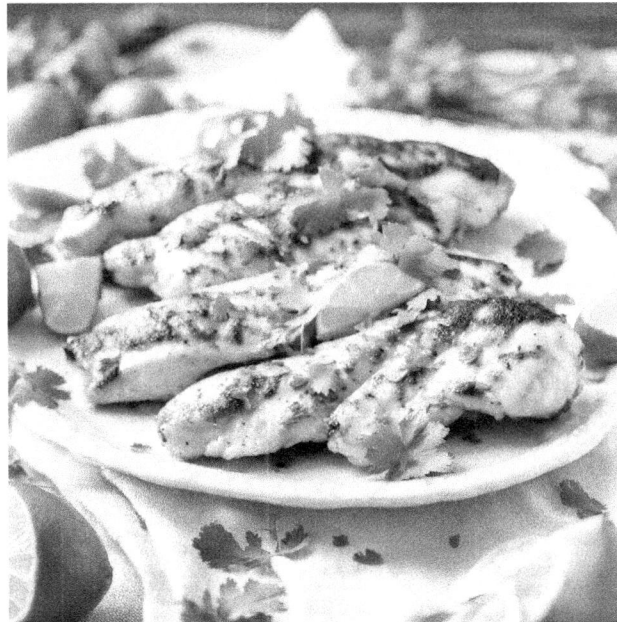

15. Chicken and Sweet Potato Skillet

Servings: 4

Cooking Time: 30 minutes

Ingredients:

- 1 pound boneless, skinless chicken breasts, cut into bite-sized pieces
- 2 tablespoons olive oil
- 2 medium sweet potatoes, peeled and diced
- 1 red bell pepper, diced
- 1 yellow bell pepper, diced
- 1 small onion, diced
- 3 cloves garlic, minced
- 1 teaspoon dried thyme
- 1/4 cup low-sodium chicken broth

Instructions:

1. Heat 1 tablespoon of olive oil in a large skillet over medium-high heat.
2. Add the chicken pieces and cook for about 5-6 minutes until browned and cooked through. Remove the chicken from the skillet and set aside.
3. In the same skillet, add the remaining tablespoon of olive oil.
4. Add the sweet potatoes, bell peppers, and onion. Cook for about 10-12 minutes until the vegetables are tender.
5. Add the garlic and thyme and cook for another 1-2 minutes.
6. Return the chicken to the skillet and add the chicken broth. Stir to combine and cook for another 2-3 minutes until heated through.
7. Serve immediately.

Nutritional Information (per serving):

- Calories: 320
- Protein: 28g
- Carbohydrates: 28g
- Dietary Fiber: 6g
- Sugars: 8g
- Fat: 12g
- Saturated Fat: 2g
- Sodium: 150mg

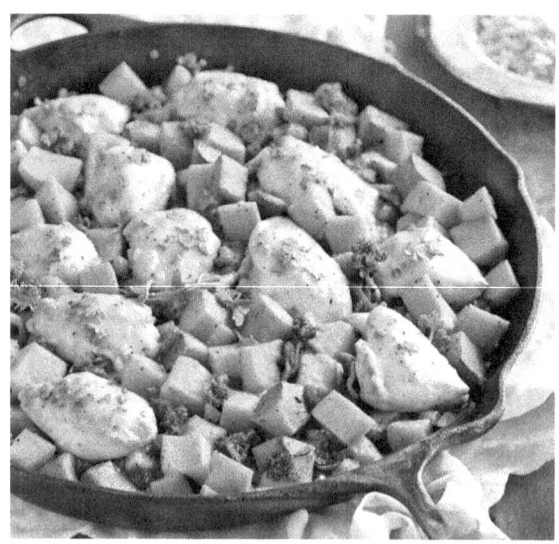

16. Chicken and Lentil Stew

Servings: 4

Cooking Time: 45 minutes

Ingredients:

- 1 pound boneless, skinless chicken thighs, cut into bite-sized pieces
- 2 tablespoons olive oil
- 1 onion, diced
- 3 cloves garlic, minced
- 2 carrots, sliced
- 2 celery stalks, sliced
- 1 cup dried lentils, rinsed
- 4 cups low-sodium chicken broth
- 1 teaspoon dried thyme
- 1 teaspoon ground cumin
- 1/4 cup fresh parsley, chopped

Instructions:

1. Heat the olive oil in a large pot over medium-high heat.
2. Add the chicken pieces and cook for about 5-6 minutes until browned and cooked through. Remove the chicken from the pot and set aside.
3. In the same pot, add the onion, garlic, carrots, and celery. Cook for about 5-6 minutes until the vegetables are softened.
4. Add the lentils, chicken broth, thyme, and cumin to the pot. Bring to a boil.
5. Reduce the heat to low, cover, and simmer for about 25-30 minutes until the lentils are tender.
6. Return the chicken to the pot and stir to combine. Cook for another 5 minutes until heated through.
7. Garnish with fresh parsley and serve immediately.

Nutritional Information (per serving):

- Calories: 350
- Protein: 32g
- Carbohydrates: 30g
- Dietary Fiber: 10g
- Sugars: 6g
- Fat: 12g
- Saturated Fat: 2.5g
- Sodium: 300mg

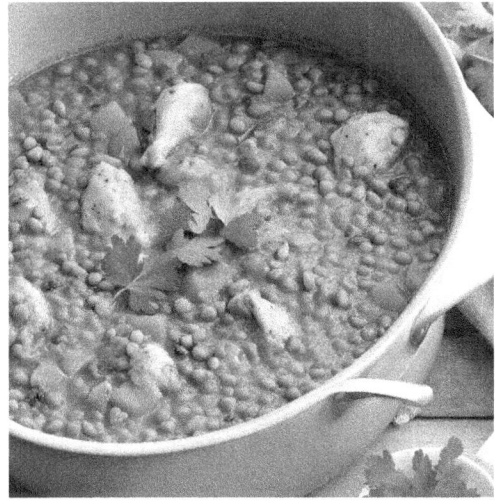

17. Chicken and Chickpea Salad

Servings: 4

Cooking Time: 20 minutes

Ingredients:

- 1 pound boneless, skinless chicken breasts, grilled and sliced
- 1 can (15 ounces) chickpeas, drained and rinsed
- 1 cucumber, diced
- 1 red bell pepper, diced
- 1/4 cup red onion, finely chopped
- 1/4 cup fresh parsley, chopped
- 2 tablespoons olive oil
- 2 tablespoons fresh lemon juice
- 1 teaspoon ground cumin

Instructions:

1. In a large bowl, combine the grilled chicken, chickpeas, cucumber, red bell pepper, red onion, and parsley.
2. In a small bowl, whisk together the olive oil, lemon juice, and cumin.
3. Pour the dressing over the salad and toss to combine.
4. Serve immediately.

Nutritional Information (per serving):

- Calories: 320
- Protein: 32g
- Carbohydrates: 25g
- Dietary Fiber: 7g
- Sugars: 3g
- Fat: 12g
- Saturated Fat: 1.5g
- Sodium: 220mg

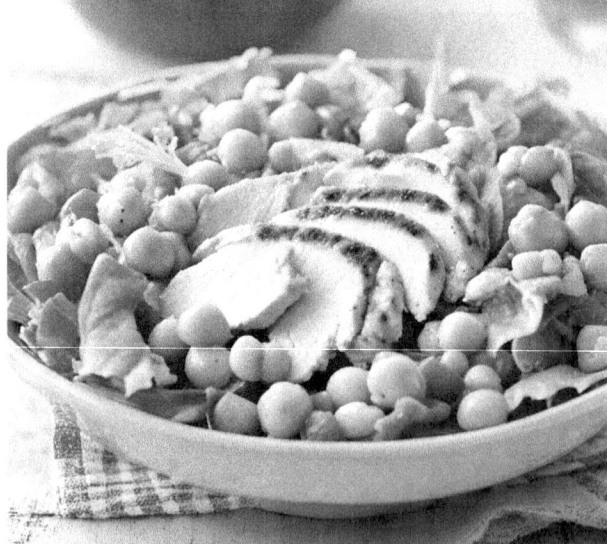

18. Chicken and Vegetable Soup

Servings: 4
Cooking Time: 40 minutes
Ingredients:

- 1 pound boneless, skinless chicken breasts, cubed
- 2 tablespoons olive oil
- 1 onion, diced
- 3 cloves garlic, minced
- 3 carrots, sliced
- 2 celery stalks, sliced
- 1 zucchini, diced
- 6 cups low-sodium chicken broth
- 1 teaspoon dried thyme
- 1 teaspoon dried oregano
- 1/4 cup fresh parsley, chopped

Instructions:

1. Heat the olive oil in a large pot over medium-high heat.
2. Add the chicken and cook for about 5-6 minutes until browned and cooked through. Remove the chicken and set aside.
3. In the same pot, add the onion, garlic, carrots, and celery. Cook for about 5-6 minutes until softened.
4. Add the zucchini, chicken broth, thyme, and oregano. Bring to a boil.
5. Reduce the heat to low, cover, and simmer for about 20 minutes.
6. Return the chicken to the pot and stir to combine. Cook for another 5 minutes until heated through.
7. Garnish with fresh parsley and serve immediately.

Nutritional Information (per serving):

- Calories: 250
- Protein: 28g
- Carbohydrates: 15g
- Dietary Fiber: 4g
- Sugars: 6g
- Fat: 10g
- Saturated Fat: 2g
- Sodium: 200mg

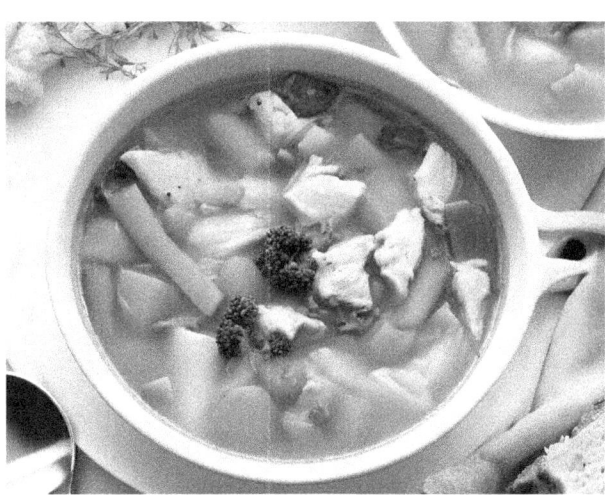

19. Chicken and Mushroom Stir-Fry

Servings: 4

Cooking Time: 20 minutes

Ingredients:

- 1 pound boneless, skinless chicken breasts, sliced
- 2 tablespoons olive oil
- 2 cups mushrooms, sliced
- 1 red bell pepper, sliced
- 1 yellow bell pepper, sliced
- 3 cloves garlic, minced
- 2 tablespoons soy sauce (low sodium)
- 1 tablespoon oyster sauce
- 1 tablespoon fresh ginger, grated
- 1/4 cup green onions, sliced

Instructions:

1. Heat the olive oil in a large skillet or wok over medium-high heat.
2. Add the chicken and cook for about 5-6 minutes until browned and cooked through. Remove the chicken from the skillet and set aside.
3. In the same skillet, add the garlic and ginger, and sauté for about 1 minute until fragrant.
4. Add the mushrooms and bell peppers and stir-fry for about 5-6 minutes until the vegetables are tender-crisp.
5. In a small bowl, mix the soy sauce and oyster sauce.
6. Return the chicken to the skillet and pour the sauce mixture over the chicken and vegetables. Stir to combine and cook for another 2-3 minutes until heated through.
7. Garnish with sliced green onions and serve immediately.

Nutritional Information (per serving):

- **Calories: 280**
- Protein: 28g
- Carbohydrates: 12g
- Dietary Fiber: 3g
- Sugars: 5g
- Fat: 12g
- Saturated Fat: 2g
- Sodium: 350mg

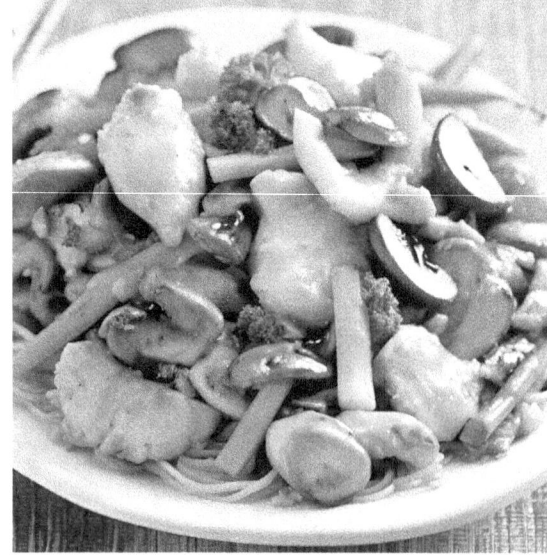

20. Chicken and Black Bean Salad

Servings: 4
Cooking Time: 20 minutes
Ingredients:

- 1 pound boneless, skinless chicken breasts, grilled and sliced
- 1 can (15 ounces) black beans, drained and rinsed
- 1 cup corn kernels (fresh or frozen)
- 1 red bell pepper, diced
- 1/4 cup red onion, finely chopped
- 1/4 cup fresh cilantro, chopped
- 2 tablespoons olive oil
- 2 tablespoons fresh lime juice
- 1 teaspoon ground cumin

Instructions:

1. In a large bowl, combine the grilled chicken, black beans, corn, red bell pepper, red onion, and cilantro.
2. In a small bowl, whisk together the olive oil, lime juice, and cumin.
3. Pour the dressing over the salad and toss to combine.
4. Serve immediately.

Nutritional Information (per serving):

- Calories: 350
- Protein: 32g
- Carbohydrates: 28g
- Dietary Fiber: 9g
- Sugars: 4g
- Fat: 14g
- Saturated Fat: 2g
- Sodium: 220mg

21. Chicken and Brussels Sprouts Skillet

Servings: 4

Cooking Time: 30 minutes

Ingredients:

- 1 pound boneless, skinless chicken breasts, cubed
- 2 tablespoons olive oil
- 4 cups Brussels sprouts, halved
- 1 red onion, sliced
- 3 cloves garlic, minced
- 1/4 cup low-sodium chicken broth
- 1 tablespoon balsamic vinegar
- 1 teaspoon dried thyme

Instructions:

1. Heat 1 tablespoon of olive oil in a large skillet over medium-high heat.
2. Add the chicken and cook for about 5-6 minutes until browned and cooked through. Remove the chicken from the skillet and set aside.
3. In the same skillet, add the remaining tablespoon of olive oil.
4. Add the Brussels sprouts and red onion. Cook for about 10-12 minutes until the vegetables are tender.
5. Add the garlic and thyme and cook for another 1-2 minutes.
6. Return the chicken to the skillet and add the chicken broth and balsamic vinegar. Stir to combine and cook for another 2-3 minutes until heated through.
7. Serve immediately.

Nutritional Information (per serving):

- Calories: 300
- Protein: 28g
- Carbohydrates: 16g
- Dietary Fiber: 6g
- Sugars: 6g
- Fat: 12g
- Saturated Fat: 2g
- Sodium: 200mg

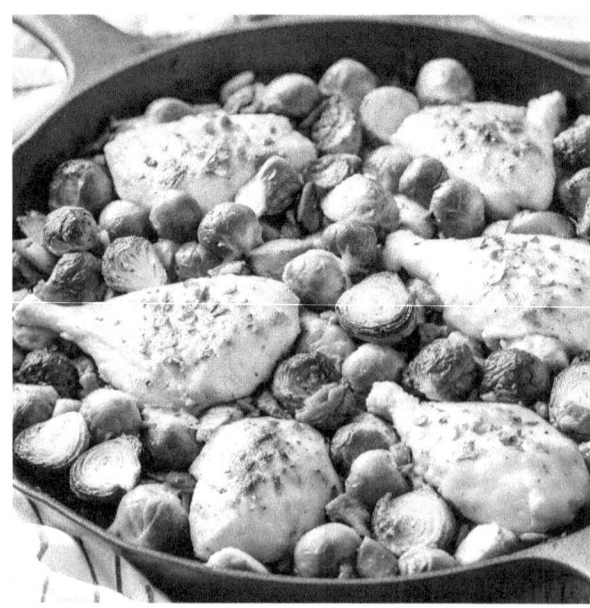

22. Chicken and Green Bean Stir-Fry

Servings: 4

Cooking Time: 20 minutes

Ingredients:

- 1 pound boneless, skinless chicken breasts, sliced
- 2 tablespoons olive oil
- 2 cups green beans, trimmed
- 1 red bell pepper, sliced
- 1 yellow bell pepper, sliced
- 3 cloves garlic, minced
- 1 tablespoon fresh ginger, grated
- 2 tablespoons soy sauce (low sodium)
- 1 tablespoon sesame oil
- 1/4 cup green onions, sliced

Instructions:

1. Heat the olive oil in a large skillet or wok over medium-high heat.
2. Add the chicken and cook for about 5-6 minutes until browned and cooked through. Remove the chicken from the skillet and set aside.
3. In the same skillet, add the garlic and ginger, and sauté for about 1 minute until fragrant.
4. Add the green beans and bell peppers and stir-fry for about 5-6 minutes until the vegetables are tender-crisp.
5. In a small bowl, mix the soy sauce and sesame oil.
6. Return the chicken to the skillet and pour the soy sauce mixture over the chicken and vegetables. Stir to combine and cook for another 2-3 minutes until heated through.
7. Garnish with sliced green onions and serve immediately.

Nutritional Information (per serving):

- Calories: 260
- Protein: 28g
- Carbohydrates: 10g
- Dietary Fiber: 4g
- Sugars: 4g
- Fat: 12g
- Saturated Fat: 2g
- Sodium: 320mg

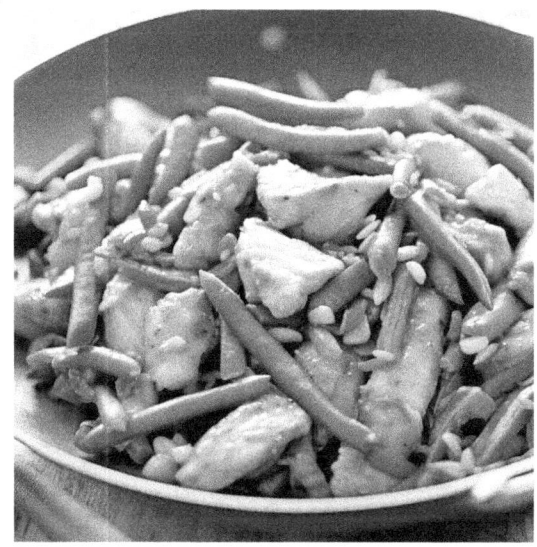

23. Chicken and Pineapple Skewers

Servings: 4

Cooking Time: 30 minutes

Ingredients:

- 1 pound boneless, skinless chicken breasts, cut into 1-inch cubes
- 2 cups fresh pineapple chunks
- 1 red bell pepper, cut into 1-inch pieces
- 1 yellow bell pepper, cut into 1-inch pieces
- 2 tablespoons olive oil
- 2 tablespoons soy sauce (low sodium)
- 1 tablespoon honey
- 1 tablespoon fresh lime juice
- 1 teaspoon ground cumin

Instructions:

1. In a large bowl, mix the olive oil, soy sauce, honey, lime juice, and cumin.
2. Add the chicken cubes to the bowl and toss to coat. Marinate for at least 30 minutes in the refrigerator.
3. Preheat the grill to medium-high heat.
4. Thread the chicken, pineapple, and bell peppers alternately onto skewers.
5. Grill the skewers for about 10-12 minutes, turning occasionally, until the chicken is cooked through and the vegetables are tender.
6. Serve immediately.

Nutritional Information (per serving):

- Calories: 300
- Protein: 28g
- Carbohydrates: 20g
- Dietary Fiber: 3g
- Sugars: 15g
- Fat: 12g
- Saturated Fat: 2g
- Sodium: 320mg

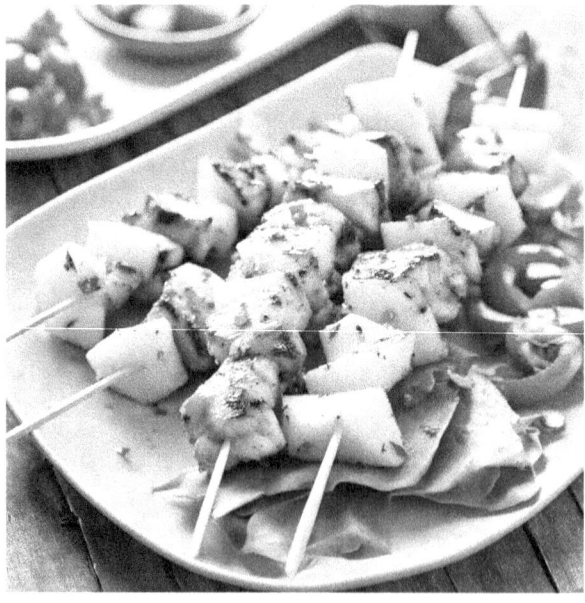

24. Chicken and Zucchini Noodles

Servings: 4
Cooking Time: 20 minutes
Ingredients:

- 1 pound boneless, skinless chicken breasts, sliced
- 2 tablespoons olive oil
- 3 zucchinis, spiralized into noodles
- 1 red bell pepper, sliced
- 1 yellow bell pepper, sliced
- 3 cloves garlic, minced
- 1 tablespoon fresh lemon juice
- 1 teaspoon dried oregano
- 1/4 cup grated Parmesan cheese (optional)

Instructions:

1. Heat the olive oil in a large skillet over medium-high heat.
2. Add the chicken and cook for about 5-6 minutes until browned and cooked through. Remove the chicken from the skillet and set aside.
3. In the same skillet, add the garlic and sauté for about 1 minute until fragrant.
4. Add the bell peppers and cook for about 3-4 minutes until tender.
5. Add the zucchini noodles, lemon juice, and oregano. Cook for another 2-3 minutes until the zucchini noodles are tender.
6. Return the chicken to the skillet and stir to combine. Cook for another 2 minutes until heated through.
7. Sprinkle with grated Parmesan cheese (if using) and serve immediately.

Nutritional Information (per serving):

- Calories: 260
- Protein: 28g
- Carbohydrates: 10g
- Dietary Fiber: 3g
- Sugars: 6g
- Fat: 12g
- Saturated Fat: 2g
- Sodium: 220mg

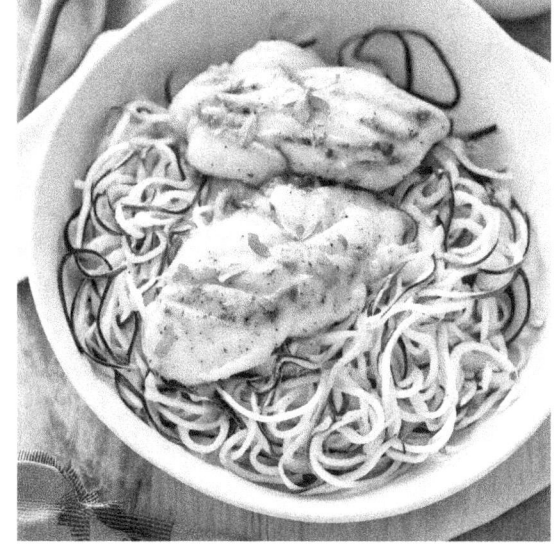

Soup and Stew Recipes

1. Lentil and Vegetable Stew
Servings: 6
Cooking Time: 50 minutes
Ingredients:

- 1 cup green or brown lentils, rinsed
- 2 tablespoons olive oil
- 1 onion, diced
- 3 cloves garlic, minced
- 3 carrots, sliced
- 2 celery stalks, sliced
- 1 zucchini, diced
- 1 red bell pepper, diced
- 1 can (14.5 ounces) diced tomatoes
- 6 cups low-sodium vegetable broth
- 1 teaspoon dried thyme
- 1 teaspoon dried oregano
- 1/2 teaspoon cumin
- 1/4 cup fresh parsley, chopped

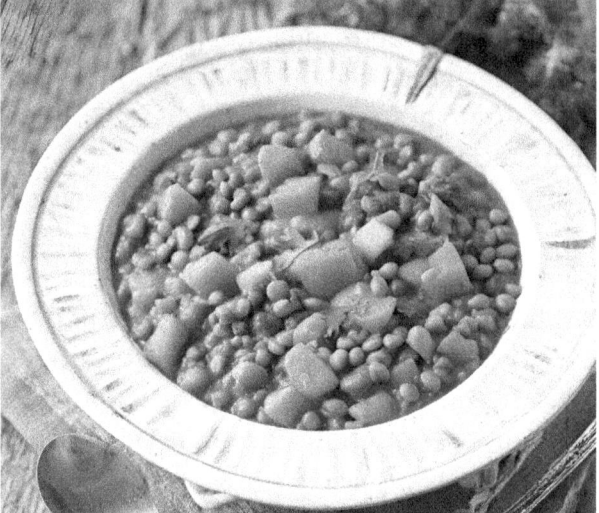

Instructions:

1. Heat the olive oil in a large pot over medium-high heat.
2. Add the onion and garlic, and sauté for about 5 minutes until softened.
3. Add the carrots, celery, zucchini, and red bell pepper. Cook for another 5 minutes until the vegetables begin to soften.
4. Stir in the lentils, diced tomatoes, vegetable broth, thyme, oregano, and cumin.
5. Bring to a boil, then reduce the heat to low and simmer for about 30-35 minutes until the lentils are tender.
6. Stir in the fresh parsley and serve immediately.

Nutritional Information (per serving):

- Calories: 250 Protein: 10g Carbohydrates: 38g   Dietary Fiber: 14g
- Sugars: 8g
- Fat: 7g
- Saturated Fat: 1g
- Sodium: 300mg

2. Quinoa and Kale Soup

Servings: 6
Cooking Time: 40 minutes
Ingredients:

- 1 cup quinoa, rinsed
- 2 tablespoons olive oil
- 1 onion, diced
- 3 cloves garlic, minced
- 3 carrots, sliced
- 2 celery stalks, sliced
- 6 cups low-sodium vegetable broth
- 1 can (14.5 ounces) diced tomatoes
- 1 teaspoon dried thyme
- 1 teaspoon dried oregano
- 4 cups chopped kale
- 1/4 cup fresh parsley, chopped

Instructions:

1. Heat the olive oil in a large pot over medium-high heat.
2. Add the onion and garlic, and sauté for about 5 minutes until softened.
3. Add the carrots and celery, and cook for another 5 minutes until the vegetables begin to soften.
4. Stir in the quinoa, vegetable broth, diced tomatoes, thyme, and oregano.
5. Bring to a boil, then reduce the heat to low and simmer for about 20 minutes until the quinoa is cooked.
6. Add the kale and cook for another 5 minutes until the kale is tender.
7. Stir in the fresh parsley and serve immediately.

Nutritional Information (per serving):

- Calories: 220
- Protein: 8g
- Carbohydrates: 34g
- Dietary Fiber: 6g
- Sugars: 7g
- Fat: 7g
- Saturated Fat: 1g
- Sodium: 250mg

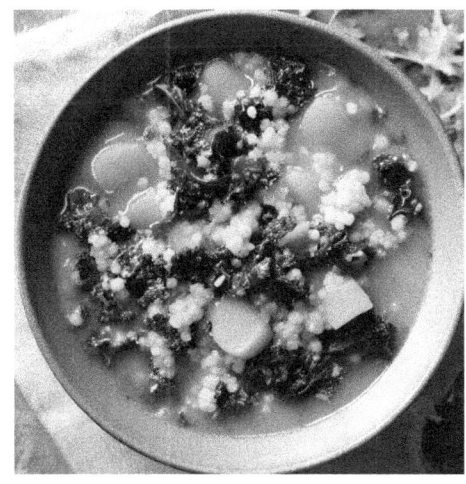

3. Carrot Ginger Soup

Servings: 4
Cooking Time: 30 minutes
Ingredients:

- 2 tablespoons olive oil
- 1 onion, diced
- 2 pounds carrots, peeled and sliced
- 1 tablespoon fresh ginger, grated
- 4 cups low-sodium vegetable broth
- 1/2 teaspoon ground cumin
- 1/4 cup coconut milk (optional)
- 1/4 cup fresh cilantro, chopped

Instructions:

1. Heat the olive oil in a large pot over medium-high heat.
2. Add the onion and sauté for about 5 minutes until softened.
3. Add the carrots and ginger, and cook for another 5 minutes.
4. Stir in the vegetable broth and cumin.
5. Bring to a boil, then reduce the heat to low and simmer for about 20 minutes until the carrots are tender.
6. Use an immersion blender to puree the soup until smooth. Alternatively, transfer the soup in batches to a blender and puree until smooth.
7. Stir in the coconut milk (if using) and heat through.
8. Garnish with fresh cilantro and serve immediately.

Nutritional Information (per serving):

- Calories: 180
- Protein: 2g
- Carbohydrates: 25g
- Dietary Fiber: 6g
- Sugars: 12g
- Fat: 9g
- Saturated Fat: 2g
- Sodium: 200mg

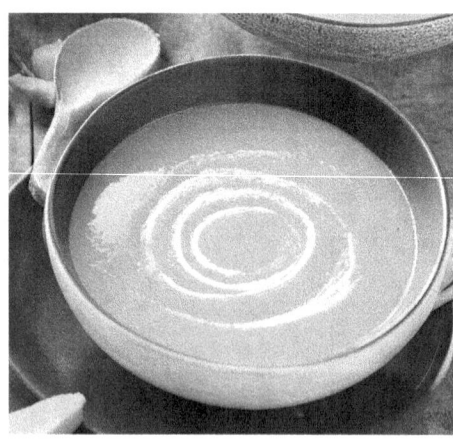

4. Minestrone Soup

Servings: 6
Cooking Time: 45 minutes
Ingredients:

- 2 tablespoons olive oil
- 1 onion, diced
- 3 cloves garlic, minced
- 2 carrots, sliced
- 2 celery stalks, sliced
- 1 zucchini, diced
- 1 cup green beans, chopped
- 1 can (14.5 ounces) diced tomatoes
- 6 cups low-sodium vegetable broth
- 1 can (15 ounces) cannellini beans, drained and rinsed
- 1 teaspoon dried oregano
- 1 teaspoon dried basil
- 1/2 cup small pasta (such as ditalini or elbow macaroni)
- 1/4 cup fresh parsley, chopped

Instructions:

1. Heat the olive oil in a large pot over medium-high heat.
2. Add the onion and garlic, and sauté for about 5 minutes until softened.
3. Add the carrots, celery, zucchini, and green beans. Cook for another 5 minutes until the vegetables begin to soften.
4. Stir in the diced tomatoes, vegetable broth, cannellini beans, oregano, and basil.
5. Bring to a boil, then reduce the heat to low and simmer for about 20 minutes.
6. Add the pasta and cook for another 10 minutes until the pasta is tender.
7. Stir in the fresh parsley and serve immediately.

Nutritional Information (per serving):

- Calories: 250
- Protein: 10g
- Carbohydrates: 40g
- Dietary Fiber: 8g
- Sugars: 7g
- Fat: 7g
- Saturated Fat: 1g
- Sodium: 250mg

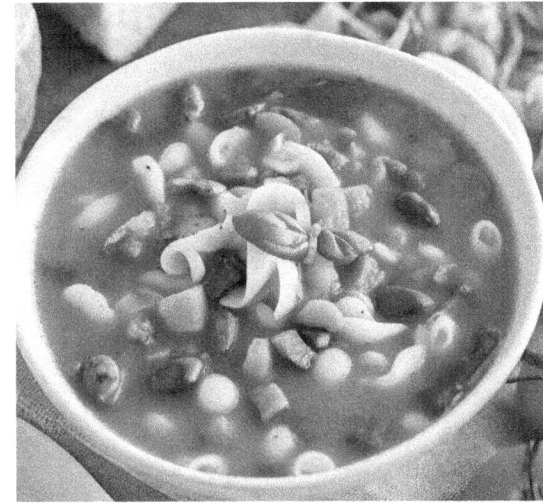

5. Tomato Basil Soup

Servings: 4
Cooking Time: 30 minutes
Ingredients:

- 2 tablespoons olive oil
- 1 onion, diced
- 3 cloves garlic, minced
- 4 cups diced tomatoes (fresh or canned)
- 4 cups low-sodium vegetable broth
- 1 teaspoon dried basil
- 1/2 teaspoon dried oregano
- 1/4 cup fresh basil, chopped
- 1/4 cup coconut milk (optional)

Instructions:

1. Heat the olive oil in a large pot over medium-high heat.
2. Add the onion and garlic, and sauté for about 5 minutes until softened.
3. Add the diced tomatoes, vegetable broth, dried basil, and oregano.
4. Bring to a boil, then reduce the heat to low and simmer for about 20 minutes.
5. Use an immersion blender to puree the soup until smooth. Alternatively, transfer the soup in batches to a blender and puree until smooth.
6. Stir in the coconut milk (if using) and heat through.
7. Garnish with fresh basil and serve immediately.

Nutritional Information (per serving):

- Calories: 180
- Protein: 3g
- Carbohydrates: 20g
- Dietary Fiber: 5g
- Sugars: 12g
- Fat: 10g
- Saturated Fat: 2g
- Sodium: 250mg

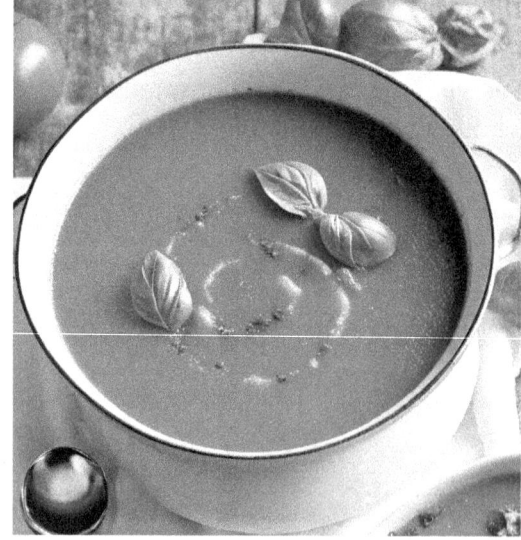

6. Spinach and White Bean Soup
Servings: 4
Cooking Time: 30 minutes
Ingredients:
- 2 tablespoons olive oil
- 1 onion, diced
- 3 cloves garlic, minced
- 4 cups low-sodium vegetable broth
- 1 can (15 ounces) white beans, drained and rinsed
- 4 cups fresh spinach, chopped
- 1 teaspoon dried thyme
- 1/4 cup fresh parsley, chopped

Instructions:
1. Heat the olive oil in a large pot over medium-high heat.
2. Add the onion and garlic, and sauté for about 5 minutes until softened.
3. Add the vegetable broth, white beans, and thyme. Bring to a boil.
4. Reduce the heat to low and simmer for about 10 minutes.
5. Add the chopped spinach and cook for another 5 minutes until the spinach is wilted.
6. Stir in the fresh parsley and serve immediately.

Nutritional Information (per serving):
- Calories: 200
- Protein: 8g
- Carbohydrates: 25g
- Dietary Fiber: 8g
- Sugars: 4g
- Fat: 8g
- Saturated Fat: 1g
- Sodium: 200mg

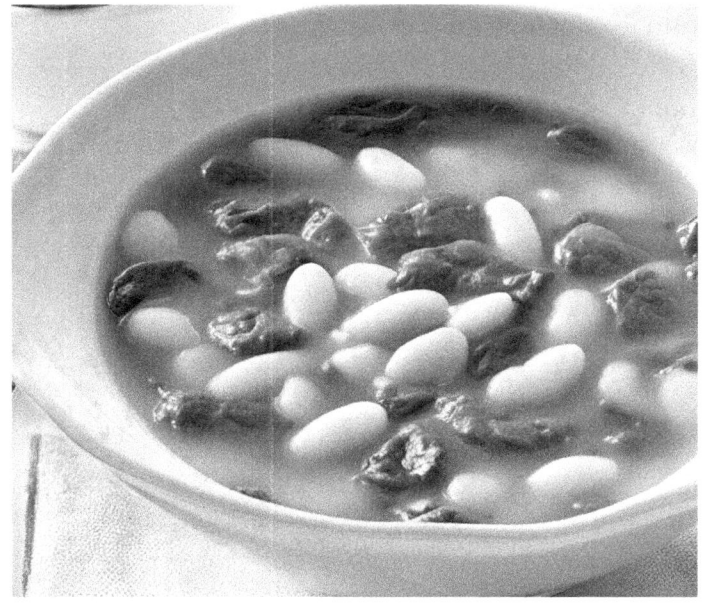

7. Sweet Potato and Black Bean Stew

Servings: 6
Cooking Time: 45 minutes
Ingredients:

- 2 tablespoons olive oil
- 1 onion, diced
- 3 cloves garlic, minced
- 2 large sweet potatoes, peeled and cubed
- 1 red bell pepper, diced
- 1 can (15 ounces) black beans, drained and rinsed
- 4 cups low-sodium vegetable broth
- 1 can (14.5 ounces) diced tomatoes
- 1 teaspoon ground cumin
- 1 teaspoon chili powder
- 1/4 cup fresh cilantro, chopped

Instructions:

1. Heat the olive oil in a large pot over medium-high heat.
2. Add the onion and garlic, and sauté for about 5 minutes until softened.
3. Add the sweet potatoes and red bell pepper, and cook for another 5 minutes.
4. Stir in the black beans, vegetable broth, diced tomatoes, cumin, and chili powder.
5. Bring to a boil, then reduce the heat to low and simmer for about 25-30 minutes until the sweet potatoes are tender.
6. Stir in the fresh cilantro and serve immediately.

Nutritional Information (per serving):

- Calories: 280
- Protein: 8g
- Carbohydrates: 50g
- Dietary Fiber: 12g
- Sugars: 12g
- Fat: 8g
- Saturated Fat: 1g
- Sodium: 220mg

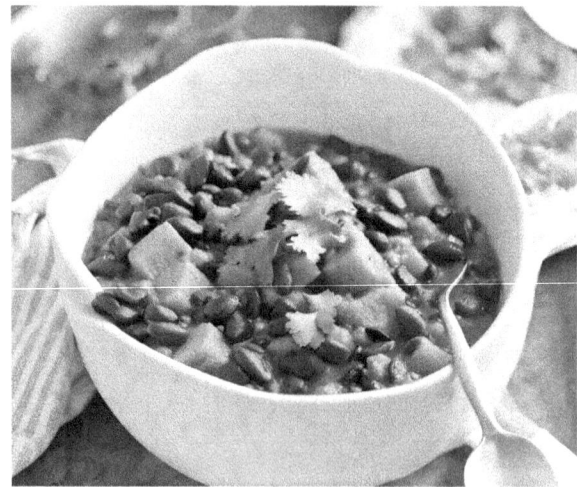

8. Vegetable Barley Soup

Servings: 6
Cooking Time: 60 minutes
Ingredients:

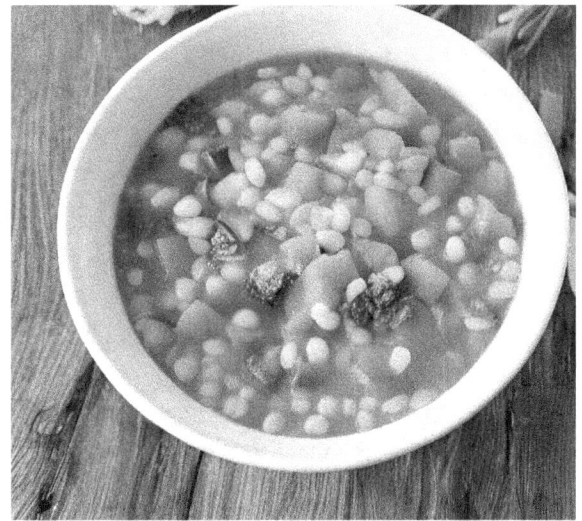

- 1 cup pearl barley
- 2 tablespoons olive oil
- 1 onion, diced
- 3 cloves garlic, minced
- 3 carrots, sliced
- 2 celery stalks, sliced
- 1 zucchini, diced
- 1 red bell pepper, diced
- 1 can (14.5 ounces) diced tomatoes
- 6 cups low-sodium vegetable broth
- 1 teaspoon dried thyme
- 1 teaspoon dried oregano
- 1/4 cup fresh parsley, chopped

Instructions:

1. Rinse the barley under cold water.
2. Heat the olive oil in a large pot over medium-high heat.
3. Add the onion and garlic, and sauté for about 5 minutes until softened.
4. Add the carrots, celery, zucchini, and red bell pepper. Cook for another 5 minutes.
5. Stir in the barley, diced tomatoes, vegetable broth, thyme, and oregano.
6. Bring to a boil, then reduce the heat to low and simmer for about 45 minutes until the barley is tender.
7. Stir in the fresh parsley and serve immediately.

Nutritional Information (per serving):

- Calories: 250
- Protein: 6g
- Carbohydrates: 45g
- Dietary Fiber: 10g
- Sugars: 10g
- Fat: 7g
- Saturated Fat: 1g
- Sodium: 220mg

9. Broccoli and Cauliflower Soup

Servings: 4

Cooking Time: 30 minutes

Ingredients:

- 2 tablespoons olive oil
- 1 onion, diced
- 3 cloves garlic, minced
- 4 cups broccoli florets
- 4 cups cauliflower florets
- 4 cups low-sodium vegetable broth
- 1 teaspoon dried thyme
- 1/2 cup unsweetened almond milk (optional)
- 1/4 cup fresh parsley, chopped

Instructions:

1. Heat the olive oil in a large pot over medium-high heat.
2. Add the onion and garlic, and sauté for about 5 minutes until softened.
3. Add the broccoli and cauliflower, and cook for another 5 minutes.
4. Stir in the vegetable broth and thyme.
5. Bring to a boil, then reduce the heat to low and simmer for about 15 minutes until the vegetables are tender.
6. Use an immersion blender to puree the soup until smooth. Alternatively, transfer the soup in batches to a blender and puree until smooth.
7. Stir in the almond milk (if using) and heat through.
8. Garnish with fresh parsley and serve immediately.

Nutritional Information (per serving):

- Calories: 180
- Protein: 4g
- Carbohydrates: 20g
- Dietary Fiber: 8g
- Sugars: 6g
- Fat: 9g
- Saturated Fat: 1g
- Sodium: 200mg

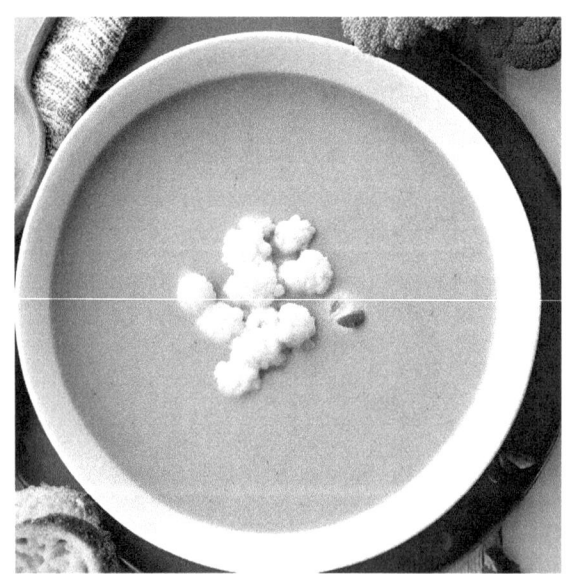

10. Beet and Carrot Soup

Servings: 4
Cooking Time: 45 minutes
Ingredients:

- 2 tablespoons olive oil
- 1 onion, diced
- 3 cloves garlic, minced
- 3 large beets, peeled and diced
- 4 carrots, sliced
- 4 cups low-sodium vegetable broth
- 1 teaspoon ground cumin
- 1/2 teaspoon ground coriander
- 1/4 cup coconut milk (optional)
- 1/4 cup fresh cilantro, chopped

Instructions:

1. Heat the olive oil in a large pot over medium-high heat.
2. Add the onion and garlic, and sauté for about 5 minutes until softened.
3. Add the beets and carrots, and cook for another 5 minutes.
4. Stir in the vegetable broth, cumin, and coriander.
5. Bring to a boil, then reduce the heat to low and simmer for about 30 minutes until the vegetables are tender.
6. Use an immersion blender to puree the soup until smooth. Alternatively, transfer the soup in batches to a blender and puree until smooth.
7. Stir in the coconut milk (if using) and heat through.
8. Garnish with fresh cilantro and serve immediately.

Nutritional Information (per serving):

- Calories: 200
- Protein: 4g
- Carbohydrates: 30g
- Dietary Fiber: 8g
- Sugars: 15g
- Fat: 9g
- Saturated Fat: 2g
- Sodium: 220mg

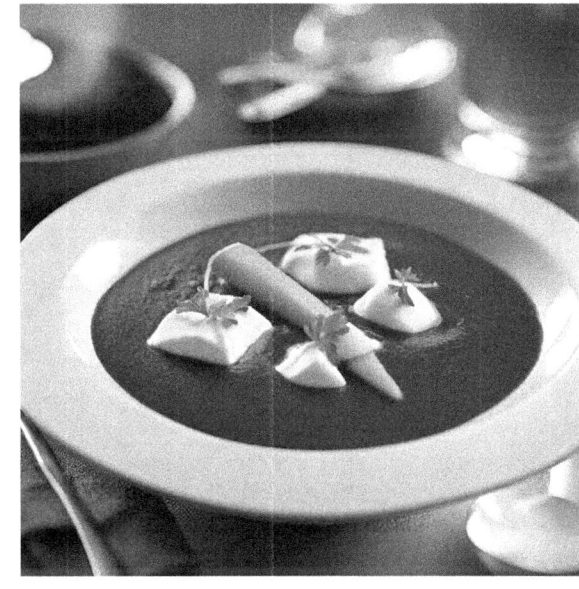

11. Zucchini and Tomato Soup

Servings: 4
Cooking Time: 30 minutes
Ingredients:

- 2 tablespoons olive oil
- 1 onion, diced
- 3 cloves garlic, minced
- 4 cups zucchini, diced
- 4 cups tomatoes, diced (fresh or canned)
- 4 cups low-sodium vegetable broth
- 1 teaspoon dried basil
- 1/2 teaspoon dried oregano
- 1/4 cup fresh basil, chopped

Instructions:

1. Heat the olive oil in a large pot over medium-high heat.
2. Add the onion and garlic, and sauté for about 5 minutes until softened.
3. Add the zucchini and tomatoes, and cook for another 5 minutes.
4. Stir in the vegetable broth, dried basil, and oregano.
5. Bring to a boil, then reduce the heat to low and simmer for about 20 minutes until the vegetables are tender.
6. Use an immersion blender to puree the soup until smooth. Alternatively, transfer the soup in batches to a blender and puree until smooth.
7. Garnish with fresh basil and serve immediately.

Nutritional Information (per serving):

- Calories: 180
- Protein: 4g
- Carbohydrates: 20g
- Dietary Fiber: 6g
- Sugars: 10g
- Fat: 9g
- Saturated Fat: 1g
- Sodium: 200mg

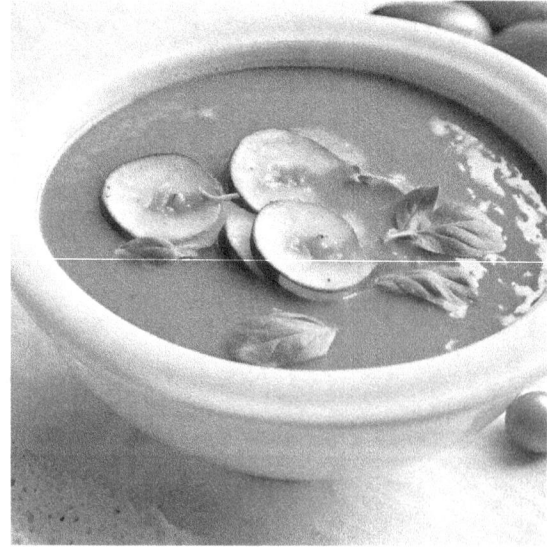

12. Kale and Potato Soup

Servings: 4

Cooking Time: 40 minutes

Ingredients:

- 2 tablespoons olive oil
- 1 onion, diced
- 3 cloves garlic, minced
- 4 cups potatoes, peeled and diced
- 4 cups low-sodium vegetable broth
- 1 teaspoon dried thyme
- 4 cups chopped kale
- 1/4 cup unsweetened almond milk (optional)

Instructions:

1. Heat the olive oil in a large pot over medium-high heat.
2. Add the onion and garlic, and sauté for about 5 minutes until softened.
3. Add the potatoes and cook for another 5 minutes.
4. Stir in the vegetable broth and thyme.
5. Bring to a boil, then reduce the heat to low and simmer for about 20 minutes until the potatoes are tender.
6. Add the kale and cook for another 5 minutes until the kale is tender.
7. Use an immersion blender to puree the soup until smooth. Alternatively, transfer the soup in batches to a blender and puree until smooth.
8. Stir in the almond milk (if using) and heat through.
9. Serve immediately.

Nutritional Information (per serving):

- Calories: 220
- Protein: 5g
- Carbohydrates: 30g
- Dietary Fiber: 6g
- Sugars: 5g
- Fat: 9g
- Saturated Fat: 1g
- Sodium: 200mg

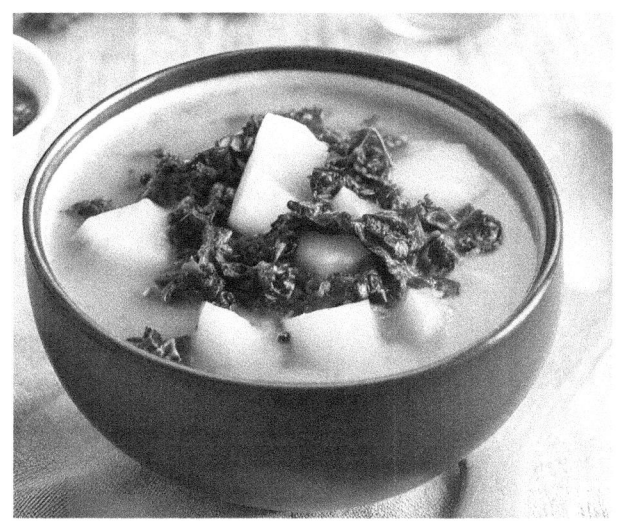

13. Mushroom and Barley Soup

Servings: 6

Cooking Time: 60 minutes

Ingredients:

- 1 cup pearl barley
- 2 tablespoons olive oil
- 1 onion, diced
- 3 cloves garlic, minced
- 2 cups mushrooms, sliced
- 3 carrots, sliced
- 2 celery stalks, sliced
- 6 cups low-sodium vegetable broth
- 1 teaspoon dried thyme
- 1/4 cup fresh parsley, chopped

Instructions:

1. Rinse the barley under cold water.
2. Heat the olive oil in a large pot over medium-high heat.
3. Add the onion and garlic, and sauté for about 5 minutes until softened.
4. Add the mushrooms, carrots, and celery. Cook for another 5 minutes.
5. Stir in the barley, vegetable broth, and thyme.
6. Bring to a boil, then reduce the heat to low and simmer for about 45 minutes until the barley is tender.
7. Stir in the fresh parsley and serve immediately.

Nutritional Information (per serving):

- Calories: 250
- Protein: 6g
- Carbohydrates: 45g
- Dietary Fiber: 10g
- Sugars: 10g
- Fat: 7g
- Saturated Fat: 1g
- Sodium: 220mg

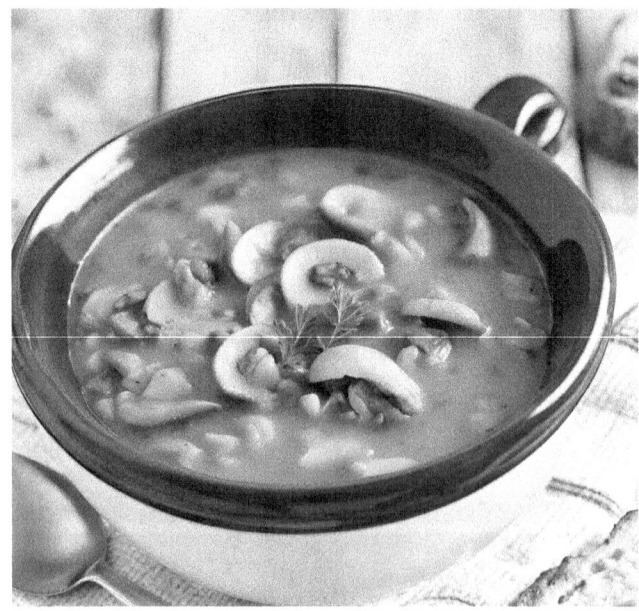

14. Pea and Mint Soup

Servings: 4
Cooking Time: 30 minutes
Ingredients:

- 2 tablespoons olive oil
- 1 onion, diced
- 3 cloves garlic, minced
- 4 cups peas (fresh or frozen)
- 4 cups low-sodium vegetable broth
- 1/4 cup fresh mint, chopped
- 1/4 cup coconut milk (optional)

Instructions:

1. Heat the olive oil in a large pot over medium-high heat.
2. Add the onion and garlic, and sauté for about 5 minutes until softened.
3. Add the peas and cook for another 5 minutes.
4. Stir in the vegetable broth and bring to a boil.
5. Reduce the heat to low and simmer for about 10 minutes until the peas are tender.
6. Use an immersion blender to puree the soup until smooth. Alternatively, transfer the soup in batches to a blender and puree until smooth.
7. Stir in the fresh mint and coconut milk (if using) and heat through.
8. Serve immediately.

Nutritional Information (per serving):

- Calories: 200
- Protein: 6g
- Carbohydrates: 30g
- Dietary Fiber: 10g
- Sugars: 10g
- Fat: 7g
- Saturated Fat: 1g
- Sodium: 200mg

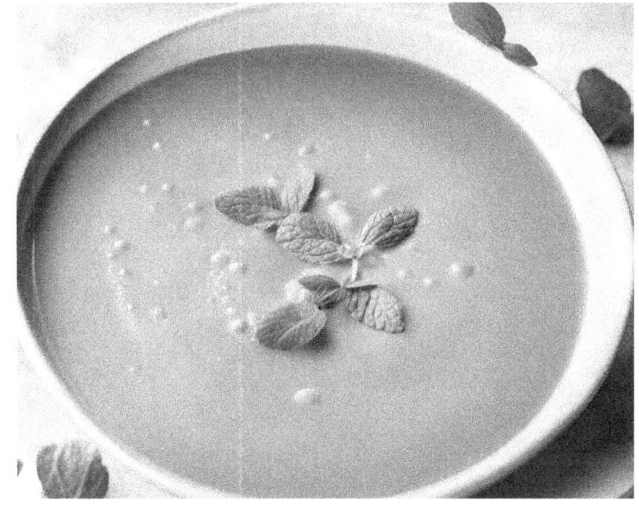

15. Carrot and Coriander Soup

Servings: 4

Cooking Time: 30 minutes

Ingredients:

- 2 tablespoons olive oil
- 1 onion, diced
- 3 cloves garlic, minced
- 6 carrots, peeled and sliced
- 4 cups low-sodium vegetable broth
- 1 teaspoon ground coriander
- 1/4 cup fresh coriander (cilantro), chopped

Instructions:

1. Heat the olive oil in a large pot over medium-high heat.
2. Add the onion and garlic, and sauté for about 5 minutes until softened.
3. Add the carrots and cook for another 5 minutes.
4. Stir in the vegetable broth and ground coriander.
5. Bring to a boil, then reduce the heat to low and simmer for about 20 minutes until the carrots are tender.
6. Use an immersion blender to puree the soup until smooth. Alternatively, transfer the soup in batches to a blender and puree until smooth.
7. Garnish with fresh coriander and serve immediately.

Nutritional Information (per serving):

- Calories: 180
- Protein: 3g
- Carbohydrates: 25g
- Dietary Fiber: 6g
- Sugars: 12g
- Fat: 9g
- Saturated Fat: 1g
- Sodium: 200mg

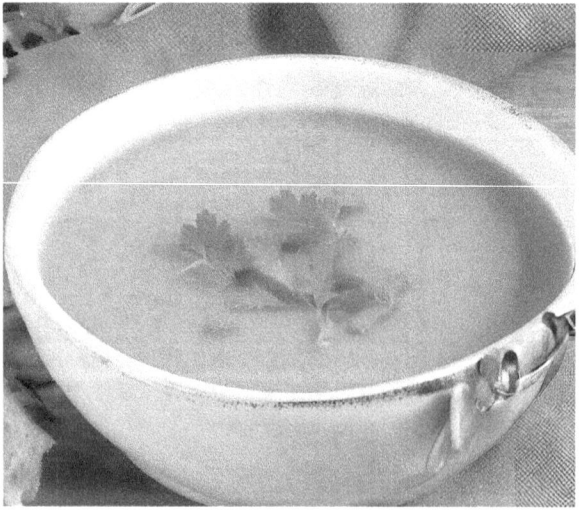

16. Tomato and Red Pepper Soup
Servings: 4
Cooking Time: 30 minutes
Ingredients:

- 2 tablespoons olive oil
- 1 onion, diced
- 3 cloves garlic, minced
- 4 large tomatoes, diced
- 2 red bell peppers, diced
- 4 cups low-sodium vegetable broth
- 1 teaspoon dried basil
- 1/4 cup coconut milk (optional)
- 1/4 cup fresh basil, chopped

Instructions:

1. Heat the olive oil in a large pot over medium-high heat.
2. Add the onion and garlic, and sauté for about 5 minutes until softened.
3. Add the tomatoes and red bell peppers, and cook for another 5 minutes.
4. Stir in the vegetable broth and dried basil.
5. Bring to a boil, then reduce the heat to low and simmer for about 20 minutes until the vegetables are tender.
6. Use an immersion blender to puree the soup until smooth. Alternatively, transfer the soup in batches to a blender and puree until smooth.
7. Stir in the coconut milk (if using) and heat through.
8. Garnish with fresh basil and serve immediately.

Nutritional Information (per serving):

- Calories: 180
- Protein: 3g
- Carbohydrates: 20g
- Dietary Fiber: 6g
- Sugars: 10g
- Fat: 9g
- Saturated Fat: 2g
- Sodium: 200mg

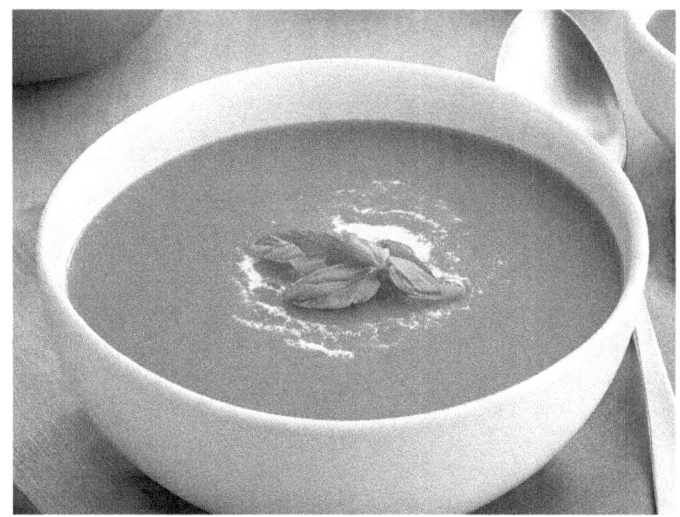

17. Broccoli and Potato Soup

Servings: 4
Cooking Time: 40 minutes
Ingredients:

- 2 tablespoons olive oil
- 1 onion, diced
- 3 cloves garlic, minced
- 4 cups broccoli florets
- 4 cups potatoes, peeled and diced
- 4 cups low-sodium vegetable broth
- 1 teaspoon dried thyme
- 1/4 cup unsweetened almond milk (optional)
- 1/4 cup fresh parsley, chopped

Instructions:

1. Heat the olive oil in a large pot over medium-high heat.
2. Add the onion and garlic, and sauté for about 5 minutes until softened.
3. Add the broccoli and potatoes, and cook for another 5 minutes.
4. Stir in the vegetable broth and thyme.
5. Bring to a boil, then reduce the heat to low and simmer for about 25 minutes until the vegetables are tender.
6. Use an immersion blender to puree the soup until smooth. Alternatively, transfer the soup in batches to a blender and puree until smooth.
7. Stir in the almond milk (if using) and heat through.
8. Garnish with fresh parsley and serve immediately.

Nutritional Information (per serving):

- Calories: 220
- Protein: 5g
- Carbohydrates: 30g
- Dietary Fiber: 6g
- Sugars: 5g
- Fat: 9g
- Saturated Fat: 1g
- Sodium: 200mg

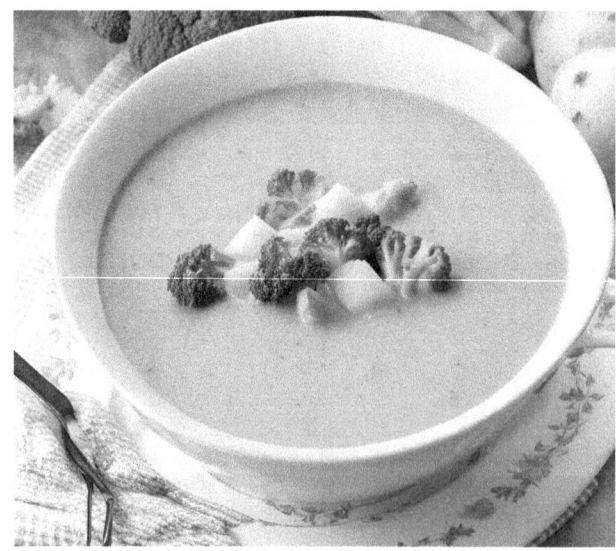

18. Pumpkin and Lentil Soup

Servings: 6
Cooking Time: 45 minutes
Ingredients:

- 2 tablespoons olive oil
- 1 onion, diced
- 3 cloves garlic, minced
- 4 cups pumpkin, peeled and diced
- 1 cup red lentils, rinsed
- 6 cups low-sodium vegetable broth
- 1 teaspoon ground cumin
- 1/2 teaspoon ground coriander
- 1/4 cup coconut milk (optional)
- 1/4 cup fresh cilantro, chopped

Instructions:

1. Heat the olive oil in a large pot over medium-high heat.
2. Add the onion and garlic, and sauté for about 5 minutes until softened.
3. Add the pumpkin and cook for another 5 minutes.
4. Stir in the lentils, vegetable broth, cumin, and coriander.
5. Bring to a boil, then reduce the heat to low and simmer for about 30 minutes until the pumpkin and lentils are tender.
6. Use an immersion blender to puree the soup until smooth. Alternatively, transfer the soup in batches to a blender and puree until smooth.
7. Stir in the coconut milk (if using) and heat through.
8. Garnish with fresh cilantro and serve immediately.

Nutritional Information (per serving):

- Calories: 240
- Protein: 8g
- Carbohydrates: 35g
- Dietary Fiber: 10g
- Sugars: 10g
- Fat: 9g
- Saturated Fat: 2g
- Sodium: 220mg

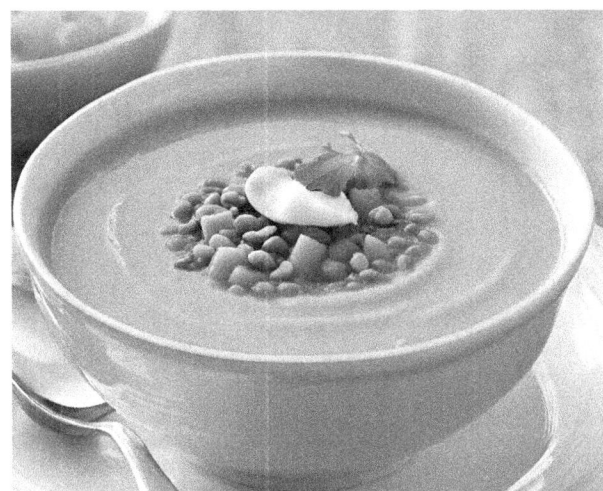

19. Carrot and Sweet Potato Soup

Servings: 4
Cooking Time: 40 minutes
Ingredients:

- 2 tablespoons olive oil
- 1 onion, diced
- 3 cloves garlic, minced
- 4 cups carrots, peeled and sliced
- 2 large sweet potatoes, peeled and diced
- 4 cups low-sodium vegetable broth
- 1 teaspoon ground ginger
- 1/2 teaspoon ground cinnamon
- 1/4 cup coconut milk (optional)
- 1/4 cup fresh cilantro, chopped

Instructions:

1. Heat the olive oil in a large pot over medium-high heat.
2. Add the onion and garlic, and sauté for about 5 minutes until softened.
3. Add the carrots and sweet potatoes, and cook for another 5 minutes.
4. Stir in the vegetable broth, ginger, and cinnamon.
5. Bring to a boil, then reduce the heat to low and simmer for about 25 minutes until the vegetables are tender.
6. Use an immersion blender to puree the soup until smooth. Alternatively, transfer the soup in batches to a blender and puree until smooth.
7. Stir in the coconut milk (if using) and heat through.
8. Garnish with fresh cilantro and serve immediately.

Nutritional Information (per serving):

- Calories: 220
- Protein: 3g
- Carbohydrates: 35g
- Dietary Fiber: 8g
- Sugars: 12g
- Fat: 9g
- Saturated Fat: 2g
- Sodium: 200mg

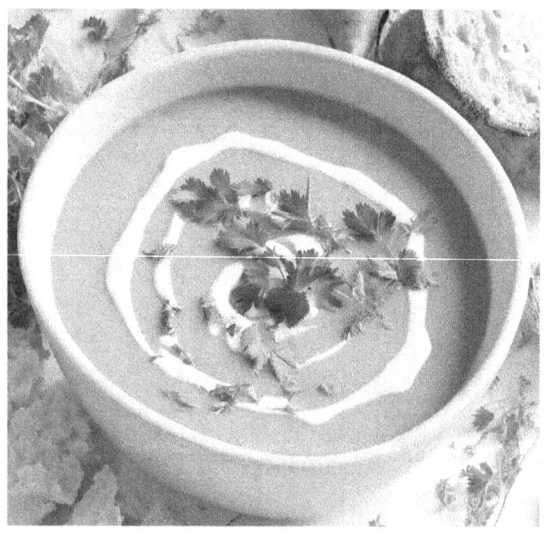

20. Zucchini and Spinach Soup
Servings: 4
Cooking Time: 30 minutes
Ingredients:

- 2 tablespoons olive oil
- 1 onion, diced
- 3 cloves garlic, minced
- 4 cups zucchini, diced
- 4 cups spinach, chopped
- 4 cups low-sodium vegetable broth
- 1 teaspoon dried basil
- 1/4 cup coconut milk (optional)
- 1/4 cup fresh parsley, chopped

Instructions:

1. Heat the olive oil in a large pot over medium-high heat.
2. Add the onion and garlic, and sauté for about 5 minutes until softened.
3. Add the zucchini and cook for another 5 minutes.
4. Stir in the vegetable broth and basil.
5. Bring to a boil, then reduce the heat to low and simmer for about 15 minutes until the zucchini is tender.
6. Add the spinach and cook for another 5 minutes until wilted.
7. Use an immersion blender to puree the soup until smooth. Alternatively, transfer the soup in batches to a blender and puree until smooth.
8. Stir in the coconut milk (if using) and heat through.
9. Garnish with fresh parsley and serve immediately.

Nutritional Information (per serving):

- Calories: 180
- Protein: 4g
- Carbohydrates: 18g
- Dietary Fiber: 6g
- Sugars: 6g
- Fat: 10g
- Saturated Fat: 2g
- Sodium: 200mg

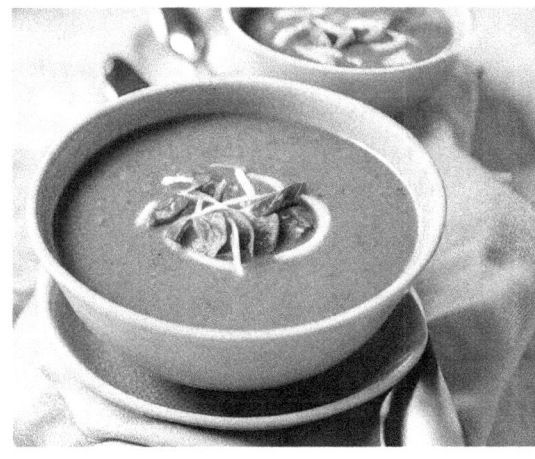

10-WEEK MEAL PLAN

Week 1

Monday
- Breakfast: Oatmeal with Fresh Berries
- Lunch: Baked Cod with Herbs
- Dinner: Chicken and Vegetable Stir-Fry

Tuesday
- Breakfast: Greek Yogurt with Honey and Nuts
- Lunch: Grilled Salmon with Lemon and Dill
- Dinner: Chicken and Broccoli Bake

Wednesday
- Breakfast: Green Smoothie
- Lunch: Steamed Tilapia with Ginger and Scallions
- Dinner: Herb Roasted Chicken

Thursday
- Breakfast: Quinoa Breakfast Bowl
- Lunch: Tuna Salad with Avocado
- Dinner: Chicken and Sweet Potato Skillet

Friday
- Breakfast: Egg White Omelet
- Lunch: Baked Mackerel with Lemon
- Dinner: Chicken and Lentil Stew

Saturday
- Breakfast: Whole Grain Pancakes
- Lunch: Fish Tacos
- Dinner: Cilantro Lime Chicken

Sunday
- Breakfast: Overnight Oats
- Lunch: Lemon Garlic Tilapia
- Dinner: Chicken and Asparagus Stir-Fry

Week 2

Monday
- Breakfast: Smoothie Bowl
- Lunch: Broiled Salmon with Asparagus
- Dinner: Chicken and Brussels Sprouts Skillet

Tuesday
- Breakfast: Buckwheat Porridge
- Lunch: Seared Scallops with Spinach
- Dinner: Chicken and Black Bean Salad

Wednesday
- Breakfast: Nut Butter and Banana on Whole Grain Bread
- Lunch: Salmon and Quinoa Bowl
- Dinner: Baked Chicken with Rosemary and Garlic

Thursday
- Breakfast: Apple Cinnamon Quinoa
- Lunch: Cod with Tomato Basil Sauce
- Dinner: Lemon Pepper Chicken

Friday
- Breakfast: Berry Parfait
- Lunch: Grilled Lemon Herb Tuna
- Dinner: Chicken and Cauliflower Rice Stir-Fry

Saturday
- Breakfast: Spinach and Feta Wrap
- Lunch: Tilapia with Mango Salsa
- Dinner: Chicken and Chickpea Salad

Sunday
- Breakfast: Zucchini Bread
- Lunch: Salmon and Sweet Potato Cakes
- Dinner: Chicken and Green Bean Stir-Fry

Week 3

Monday
- Breakfast: Pumpkin Smoothie
- Lunch: Broiled Tilapia with Fresh Salsa
- Dinner: Chicken and Vegetable Soup

Tuesday
- Breakfast: Pear and Walnut Salad
- Lunch: Garlic Butter Salmon
- Dinner: Chicken and Pineapple Skewers

Wednesday
- Breakfast: Berry Smoothie
- Lunch: Baked Sole with Lemon and Capers
- Dinner: Chicken and Mushroom Stir-Fry

Thursday
- Breakfast: Granola and Yogurt Bowl
- Lunch: Seared Ahi Tuna Salad
- Dinner: Chicken and Potato Soup

Friday
- Breakfast: Banana Nut Muffins
- Lunch: Baked Salmon with Pesto
- Dinner: Chicken and Sweet Potato Soup

Saturday
- Breakfast: Blueberry Almond Overnight Oats
- Lunch: Sesame Crusted Tuna
- Dinner: Chicken and Zucchini Noodles

Sunday
- Breakfast: Hummus and Veggie Wrap
- Lunch: Lemon Herb Grilled Tuna
- Dinner: Kale and Potato Soup

Week 4

Monday
- Breakfast: Pear and Almond Oatmeal
- Lunch: Chicken and White Bean Soup
- Dinner: Mushroom and Barley Soup

Tuesday
- Breakfast: Carrot and Orange Smoothie
- Lunch: Chicken and Lentil Soup
- Dinner: Spinach and White Bean Soup

Wednesday
- Breakfast: Almond Flour Pancakes
- Lunch: Chicken and Tomato Soup
- Dinner: Sweet Potato and Black Bean Stew

Thursday
- Breakfast: Green Smoothie
- Lunch: Chicken and Vegetable Kebabs
- Dinner: Lentil and Vegetable Stew

Friday
- Breakfast: Greek Yogurt with Honey and Nuts
- Lunch: Chicken and Quinoa Soup
- Dinner: Tomato and Red Pepper Soup

Saturday
- Breakfast: Oatmeal with Fresh Berries
- Lunch: Chicken and Kale Soup
- Dinner: Broccoli and Cauliflower Soup

Sunday
- Breakfast: Whole Grain Pancakes
- Lunch: Chicken and Zucchini Soup
- Dinner: Beet and Carrot Soup

Week 5

Monday
- Breakfast: Egg White Omelet
- Lunch: Chicken and Sweet Potato Soup
- Dinner: Carrot and Sweet Potato Soup

Tuesday
- Breakfast: Apple Cinnamon Quinoa
- Lunch: Chicken and Potato Soup
- Dinner: Zucchini and Spinach Soup

Wednesday
- Breakfast: Spinach and Feta Wrap
- Lunch: Chicken and Mushroom Soup
- Dinner: Quinoa and Kale Soup

Thursday
- Breakfast: Nut Butter and Banana on Whole Grain Bread
- Lunch: Chicken and Lentil Stew
- Dinner: Minestrone Soup

Friday
- Breakfast: Buckwheat Porridge
- Lunch: Chicken and Vegetable Soup
- Dinner: Pumpkin and Lentil Soup

Saturday
- Breakfast: Overnight Oats
- Lunch: Chicken and Broccoli Bake
- Dinner: Broccoli and Potato Soup

Sunday
- Breakfast: Smoothie Bowl
- Lunch: Chicken and Green Bean Stir-Fry
- Dinner: Carrot and Coriander Soup

Week 6

Monday
- Breakfast: Zucchini and Tomato Soup
- Lunch: Lemon Herb Grilled Tuna
- Dinner: Chicken and Sweet Potato Skillet

Tuesday
- Breakfast: Pumpkin Smoothie
- Lunch: Broiled Tilapia with Fresh Salsa
- Dinner: Chicken and Lentil Stew

Wednesday
- Breakfast: Greek Yogurt with Honey and Nuts
- Lunch: Grilled Lemon Herb Chicken
- Dinner: Sweet Potato and Black Bean Stew

Thursday
- Breakfast: Green Smoothie
- Lunch: Steamed Tilapia with Ginger and Scallions
- Dinner: Chicken and Cauliflower Rice Stir-Fry

Friday
- Breakfast: Quinoa Breakfast Bowl
- Lunch: Seared Scallops with Spinach
- Dinner: Chicken and Brussels Sprouts Skillet

Saturday
- Breakfast: Nut Butter and Banana on Whole Grain Bread
- Lunch: Salmon and Quinoa Bowl
- Dinner: Mushroom and Barley Soup

Sunday
- Breakfast: Whole Grain Pancakes
- Lunch: Cod with Tomato Basil Sauce
- Dinner: Spinach and White Bean Soup

Week 7

Monday
- Breakfast: Egg White Omelet
- Lunch: Baked Sole with Lemon and Capers
- Dinner: Chicken and Zucchini Noodles

Tuesday
- Breakfast: Overnight Oats
- Lunch: Broiled Salmon with Asparagus
- Dinner: Tomato and Red Pepper Soup

Wednesday
- Breakfast: Smoothie Bowl
- Lunch: Lemon Garlic Tilapia
- Dinner: Kale and Potato Soup

Thursday
- Breakfast: Buckwheat Porridge
- Lunch: Tuna and White Bean Salad
- Dinner: Chicken and White Bean Soup

Friday
- Breakfast: Apple Cinnamon Quinoa
- Lunch: Sesame Crusted Tuna
- Dinner: Carrot and Sweet Potato Soup

Saturday
- Breakfast: Berry Parfait
- Lunch: Grilled Lemon Herb Tuna
- Dinner: Chicken and Pineapple Skewers

Sunday
- Breakfast: Spinach and Feta Wrap
- Lunch: Lemon Dill Tuna Steaks
- Dinner: Quinoa and Kale Soup

Week 8

Monday
- Breakfast: Pear and Walnut Salad
- Lunch: Grilled Salmon with Avocado Salsa
- Dinner: Minestrone Soup

Tuesday
- Breakfast: Berry Smoothie
- Lunch: Baked Cod with Herbs
- Dinner: Chicken and Mushroom Stir-Fry

Wednesday
- Breakfast: Granola and Yogurt Bowl
- Lunch: Broiled Tilapia with Fresh Salsa
- Dinner: Carrot and Ginger Soup

Thursday
- Breakfast: Banana Nut Muffins
- Lunch: Seared Ahi Tuna Salad
- Dinner: Chicken and Broccoli Bake

Friday
- Breakfast: Blueberry Almond Overnight Oats
- Lunch: Baked Salmon with Pesto
- Dinner: Pumpkin and Lentil Soup

Saturday
- Breakfast: Hummus and Veggie Wrap
- Lunch: Steamed Tilapia with Ginger and Scallions
- Dinner: Chicken and Green Bean Stir-Fry

Sunday
- Breakfast: Pear and Almond Oatmeal
- Lunch: Lemon Garlic Tilapia
- Dinner: Sweet Potato and Black Bean Stew

Week 9

Monday
- Breakfast: Carrot and Orange Smoothie
- Lunch: Broiled Salmon with Asparagus
- Dinner: Broccoli and Cauliflower Soup

Tuesday
- Breakfast: Almond Flour Pancakes
- Lunch: Tuna Salad with Avocado
- Dinner: Chicken and Chickpea Salad

Wednesday
- Breakfast: Green Smoothie
- Lunch: Lemon Herb Grilled Tuna
- Dinner: Tomato Basil Soup

Thursday
- Breakfast: Greek Yogurt with Honey and Nuts
- Lunch: Seared Scallops with Spinach
- Dinner: Carrot and Sweet Potato Soup

Friday
- Breakfast: Oatmeal with Fresh Berries
- Lunch: Baked Mackerel with Lemon
- Dinner: Mushroom and Barley Soup

Saturday
- Breakfast: Whole Grain Pancakes
- Lunch: Fish Tacos
- Dinner: Chicken and White Bean Soup

Sunday
- Breakfast: Overnight Oats
- Lunch: Garlic Butter Salmon
- Dinner: Zucchini and Tomato Soup

Week 10

Monday
- Breakfast: Smoothie Bowl
- Lunch: Seared Ahi Tuna Salad
- Dinner: Chicken and Kale Soup

Tuesday
- Breakfast: Buckwheat Porridge
- Lunch: Baked Sole with Lemon and Capers
- Dinner: Spinach and White Bean Soup

Wednesday
- Breakfast: Nut Butter and Banana on Whole Grain Bread
- Lunch: Broiled Tilapia with Fresh Salsa
- Dinner: Lentil and Vegetable Stew

Thursday
- Breakfast: Apple Cinnamon Quinoa
- Lunch: Baked Cod with Herbs
- Dinner: Minestrone Soup

Friday
- Breakfast: Berry Parfait
- Lunch: Grilled Lemon Herb Chicken
- Dinner: Pumpkin and Lentil Soup

Saturday
- Breakfast: Spinach and Feta Wrap
- Lunch: Lemon Garlic Tilapia
- Dinner: Tomato and Red Pepper Soup

Sunday
- Breakfast: Zucchini Bread
- Lunch: Steamed Tilapia with Ginger and Scallions
- Dinner: Broccoli and Potato Soup

WEEKLY MEAL PLANNER + WORKBOOK

	BREAKFAST	LUNCH	DINNER	SNACKS
MONDAY				
TUESDAY				
WEDNESDAY				
THURSDAY				
FRIDAY				
SATURDAY				
SUNDAY				

What are your top three health goals while following the Chronic Lymphocytic Leukemia diet? How do you plan to achieve them?

....

....

....

....

....

....

WEEKLY MEAL PLANNER + WORKBOOK

	BREAKFAST	LUNCH	DINNER	SNACKS
MONDAY				
TUESDAY				
WEDNESDAY				
THURSDAY				
FRIDAY				
SATURDAY				
SUNDAY				

Are there any foods that you particularly enjoy or dislike? How can you incorporate your preferences into this diet plan?

....

....

....

....

....

....

WEEKLY MEAL PLANNER + WORKBOOK

	BREAKFAST	LUNCH	DINNER	SNACKS
MONDAY				
TUESDAY				
WEDNESDAY				
THURSDAY				
FRIDAY				
SATURDAY				
SUNDAY				

What challenges do you anticipate facing while following this diet? What strategies can you use to overcome these challenges?

....

....

....

....

....

....

WEEKLY MEAL PLANNER + WORKBOOK

	BREAKFAST	LUNCH	DINNER	SNACKS
MONDAY				
TUESDAY				
WEDNESDAY				
THURSDAY				
FRIDAY				
SATURDAY				
SUNDAY				

How do you plan to structure your meals each day to ensure you get a balanced intake of nutrients?

....

....

....

....

....

....

WEEKLY MEAL PLANNER + WORKBOOK

	BREAKFAST	LUNCH	DINNER	SNACKS
MONDAY				
TUESDAY				
WEDNESDAY				
THURSDAY				
FRIDAY				
SATURDAY				
SUNDAY				

Why is hydration important in managing Chronic Lymphocytic Leukemia? How do you plan to ensure you stay adequately hydrated throughout the day?

....

....

....

....

....

....

WEEKLY MEAL PLANNER + WORKBOOK

	BREAKFAST	LUNCH	DINNER	SNACKS
MONDAY				
TUESDAY				
WEDNESDAY				
THURSDAY				
FRIDAY				
SATURDAY				
SUNDAY				

What cooking methods do you prefer? How can you use these methods to prepare CLL-friendly meals?

....

....

....

....

....

....

WEEKLY MEAL PLANNER + WORKBOOK

	BREAKFAST	LUNCH	DINNER	SNACKS
MONDAY				
TUESDAY				
WEDNESDAY				
THURSDAY				
FRIDAY				
SATURDAY				
SUNDAY				

How do you plan to incorporate physical activity into your daily routine alongside this diet?

....

....

....

....

....

....

WEEKLY MEAL PLANNER + WORKBOOK

	BREAKFAST	LUNCH	DINNER	SNACKS
MONDAY				
TUESDAY				
WEDNESDAY				
THURSDAY				
FRIDAY				
SATURDAY				
SUNDAY				

Who can you rely on for support as you start this diet? How can they help you stay motivated and accountable?

....

....

....

....

....

....

WEEKLY MEAL PLANNER + WORKBOOK

	BREAKFAST	LUNCH	DINNER	SNACKS
MONDAY				
TUESDAY				
WEDNESDAY				
THURSDAY				
FRIDAY				
SATURDAY				
SUNDAY				

What are the major dietary changes you need to make to follow the Chronic Lymphocytic Leukemia diet? How do you plan to implement these changes gradually?

....

....

....

....

....

....

WEEKLY MEAL PLANNER + WORKBOOK

	BREAKFAST	LUNCH	DINNER	SNACKS
MONDAY				
TUESDAY				
WEDNESDAY				
THURSDAY				
FRIDAY				
SATURDAY				
SUNDAY				

What new cooking skills do you need to learn to prepare the meals in this diet plan? How will you acquire these skills?

....

....

....

....

....

....

WEEKLY MEAL PLANNER + WORKBOOK

	BREAKFAST	LUNCH	DINNER	SNACKS
MONDAY				
TUESDAY				
WEDNESDAY				
THURSDAY				
FRIDAY				
SATURDAY				
SUNDAY				

How do you plan to stick to the CLL diet when eating out at restaurants or social gatherings?

....

....

....

....

....

....

WEEKLY MEAL PLANNER + WORKBOOK

	BREAKFAST	LUNCH	DINNER	SNACKS
MONDAY				
TUESDAY				
WEDNESDAY				
THURSDAY				
FRIDAY				
SATURDAY				
SUNDAY				

What steps can you take to ensure that you maintain this diet as a long-term lifestyle change rather than a short-term solution?

....

....

....

....

....

....

Scan the QR code below to get a surprise bonus!

www.ingramcontent.com/pod-product-compliance
Lightning Source LLC
Chambersburg PA
CBHW082108220526
45472CB00009B/2091